100 Questions & Answers About Bladder Cancer

Pamela Ellsworth, MD
Chief of Urology
UMass Memorial Medical Center

Brett Carswell, MD
Division of Urology
UMass Memorial HealthCare

JONES AND BARTLETT PUBLISHERS
Sudbury, Massachusetts
BOSTON   TORONTO   LONDON   SINGAPORE

World Headquarters

Jones and Bartlett
Publishers
40 Tall Pine Drive
Sudbury, MA 01776
info@jbpub.com
www.jbpub.com

Jones and Bartlett
Publishers Canada
6339 Ormindale Way
Mississauga, ON L5V 1J2
CANADA

Jones and Bartlett
Publishers International
Barb House, Barb Mews
London W6 7PA
UK

Jones and Bartlett's books and products are available through most bookstores and online booksellers. To contact Jones and Bartlett Publishers directly, call 800-832-0034, fax 978-443-8000, or visit our website www.jbpub.com.

Substantial discounts on bulk quantities of Jones and Bartlett's publications are available to corporations, professional associations, and other qualified organizations. For details and specific discount information, contact the special sales department at Jones and Bartlett via the above contact information or send an email to specialsales@jbpub.com.

Production Credits
Executive Publisher: Christopher Davis
Production Director: Amy Rose
Associate Production Editor: Tracey Chapman
Editorial Assistant: Kathy Richardson
Marketing Associate: Laura Kavigian
Manufacturing Buyer: Therese Connell
Composition: Northeast Compositors, Inc.
Cover Design: Becky Senecal
Cover Image: © Photodisc; Photos.com
Printing and Binding: Malloy, Inc.
Cover Printing: Malloy, Inc.

Library of Congress Cataloging-in-Publication Data
Ellsworth, Pamela.
100 Q&A about bladder cancer / Pamela Ellsworth and Brett Carswell.
   p. cm.
Includes bibliographical references and index.
ISBN 0-7637-3253-2 (pbk.)
1. Bladder--Cancer--Popular works. I. Title: 100 Q & A about bladder cancer. II. Title: One hundred Q&A about bladder cancer. III. Carswell, Brett. IV. Title.
RC280.B5E456 2005
616.99'462--dc22
6048   2005005143

Printed in the United States of America
10 09 08 07 06   10 9 8 7 6 5 4 3 2

Contents

This book is dedicated to our patients with bladder cancer, both young and old, whom we have treated over the years. Their courage, triumphs, tragedies, and needs have inspired us to write this book.

There is a sudden silence when a doctor mentions the word "cancer." This silence is soon followed by a flood of emotions. These include sadness, fear, anxiety, helplessness, guilt, and frustration. Despite these overwhelming emotions, patients and their families are expected to quickly process the diagnosis and make major decisions regarding treatment. Often a 30 minute or 60 minute discussion with the doctor is all that transpires before choosing treatment, which may include major surgery. This may be an overwhelming or frightening time and many questions are never asked. Questions like how will surgery affect my sexual function? Will I be able to do the same things that I did prior to surgery? Will people know I have a urine bag? These questions often take a back seat initially to questions regarding the bigger issues at hand, such as will surgery cure me of my bladder cancer? What happens if the cancer has spread outside of my bladder? And can I live without a bladder? Many patients turn to friends, family, or the internet for information. While these sources can be helpful, they may not always be accurate and often reflect a single unique experience. This book is designed to answer the questions most commonly asked by our patients with bladder cancer. It is our hope that this book will serve as a resource for people with bladder cancer to help them better understand their disease and their treatment options.

PART ONE

The Basics

What is the bladder, and what does it do?

Can I live without my bladder?

What is cancer?

More ...

1. What is the bladder, and what does it do?

The **bladder** is the container in the body that stores urine. The other term for bladder is "vesical," which is derived from the Latin word *vesicular*. The bladder is a soft, round structure that is located in the **pelvis**. The pubic bone is in front of the bladder; the **rectum** in men or the **uterus** in women is behind the bladder. Urine drains into the bladder through an opening on each side at the bottom of the bladder. Urine is stored in the bladder until a person is ready to urinate. In order to urinate, the muscle in the bladder wall squeezes, pushing the urine out of the bladder through the **urethra**. In women, the urethra is short, only approximately 1 inch long. In men, it is much longer because it has to pass through the **prostate** and then the penis before finally opening at the tip of the penis.

In the middle of the **abdomen**, just beneath the lower ribs, are the kidneys. The kidneys filter the blood to produce urine. The urine that the kidneys produce exits the kidney through the **renal pelvis** and flows into the **ureters**. The ureters are soft, muscular tubes that are about the width of a pencil. They carry the urine from the kidneys down to bladder, where they open into the base of the bladder.

The adult bladder normally holds approximately 400 ml of urine. The bladder wall has three separate layers. The innermost layer that is in contact with the urine is a thin layer called the **urothelium**. The middle layer is made of muscle fibers that can squeeze. When the muscles contract, they increase the pressure inside the

Bladder

the hollow organ that stores and discharges urine from the body.

Pelvis

the part of the body that is framed by the hip bones.

Rectum

the last portion of the large intestine that communicates with the sigmoid colon above and the anus below.

Uterus

the muscular pelvic organ of the female reproductive system in which the fetus develops.

Urethra

the tube through which one urinates.

Prostate

a gland within the male reproductive system that is located just below the bladder surrounding part of the urethra, the canal that empties the bladder; produces a fluid that forms part of semen.

bladder, squeezing the urine out of the bladder. The outermost layer is a thin but protective layer called **serosa** (Figure 1).

The bladder has two functions. The first is the storage of urine, and the second is the emptying of urine. In an infant, the bladder constantly fills and empties without any control by the brain. During toilet training, the brain learns to control the bladder, enabling it to hold (store) the urine until a time when it is socially acceptable to urinate. Emptying is the second function that the bladder must perform. In infancy, before toilet training, this is actually the most important function of the bladder.

Although most of us take these two processes for granted, either one or both can malfunction. If the storage function fails, the bladder can become very small and contracted, holding just a tiny amount of

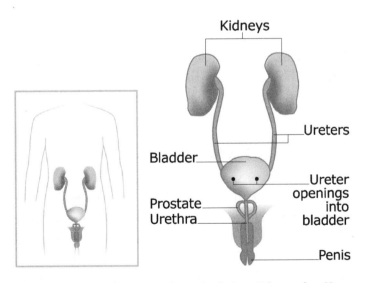

Figure 1 **The male urinary tract. Illustration by Laura Tritz, reprinted by permission from cancerfacts.com, copyright 2004.**

Abdomen

the part of the body that is below the ribs and above the pelvic bone; it contains organs such as the intestines, the liver, the kidneys, the bladder, and the prostate.

Renal pelvis

the area at the center of the kidney. Urine collects in the renal pelvis and is funneled into the ureter.

Ureters

muscular tubes that connect the kidneys to the bladder, through which urine passes into the bladder.

Urothelium

the cells lining the wall of the bladder, ureter, and the collecting system of the kidney.

The Basics

Serosa

one of the delicate
membranes of con-
nective tissue which
live the internal cavi-
ties of the body.

Urgency

the complaint of a
sudden compelling
desire to void that is
difficult to defer.

Postvoid residual

the volume of urine
left in the bladder
at the end of
micturition.

Urinary retention

the inability to uri-
nate, leading to a
filled bladder.

urine before it needs to empty. In contrast, it may become floppy and dilated, holding several liters of urine before it is ready to empty. It can also become "overactive," causing painful or annoying feelings of **urgency** between times of emptying. When the actual emptying function goes wrong, the bladder may only partially empty each time, leaving a high remaining amount of urine (the so-called **postvoid residual**). The bladder muscle may also weaken to the point where one is completely unable to urinate. This is called **urinary retention**.

When storing urine, the bladder must do so at a low pressure. This allows the new urine made in the kidneys to flow downward into the bladder. A normal bladder pressure is less than 40 cm H_2O. When the pressures are higher than this, the urine may "back up" in the kidneys. High pressures in the kidneys over a long period of time may damage the kidneys. During urination, the bladder must squeeze to force the urine out. The pressure in the bladder at these times may be much higher than 40 cm H_2O, but it does not usually damage the kidneys. This is because the pressure is elevated for just a short time and then quickly returns to normal.

2. Can I live without my bladder?

Yes. You can live without a bladder. However, you still need something that can perform the two basic functions of the bladder: storing and emptying of urine. Physicians have come up with many ways over the years to accomplish these tasks, many of which are still used today. The simplest alternative is to place drainage tubes into the kidneys that come out through the skin and connect to bags on the abdomen. These tubes are known as **nephrostomy tubes**. Nephrostomy tubes are typically inserted into a person in the X-ray department by an **interventional radiologist** who uses some light sedation. For the patient, the bag provides an easy way to store urine and can be drained several times a day when convenient by opening a small valve on the bag. These tubes can be uncomfortable, however, and may also be easily removed if tugged; therefore, they are only reasonable solutions for a short period of time or for patients who are too ill to undergo surgery. It is also possible to surgically bring the ureters directly to the skin surface (called a cutaneous **ureterostomy**). The urine then can be collected with a bag attached to the skin around the opening. Unfortunately, the ureters are relatively small, and thus any scarring or narrowing of the opening can cause a blockage of urine. This tendency to get blocked also makes cutaneous ureterostomies a poor long-term solution.

To provide a good long-term solution, surgeons most commonly use a portion of the small bowel to act as the new bladder. The identified piece of small bowel is removed from the main portion and is fashioned for its new use (see Question 79 for details). The urine that collects within this piece of bowel will ultimately be drained in one of three ways. First, the bowel can simply be left open at the skin for the urine to drain passively out into a bag that is attached to the abdomen. This type of drainage is known as a **conduit**, and the

Nephrostomy tube

a tube that is placed through the back into the kidney and allows for drainage of urine from that kidney.

Interventional radiologist

a radiologist who specializes in minimally invasive, targeted treatments performed using imagery for guidance.

Ureterostomy

surgical formation of an opening in the ureter for external drainage of the urine; in a cutaneous ureterostomy, the ureteral orifice is brought through the abdominal wall on the skin.

Conduit

a method of diverting the urine flow by sewing the ureters, the tubes that drain the kidneys, to a segment of intestine that is closed at one end. The open end is sewn to the abdominal wall to allow for urine to drain into a collecting bag.

The Basics

Urostomy

a conduit for the drainage of urine from the kidneys to the anterior abdominal wall. May be made from the small or large intestine.

Catheter

a hollow tube that allows for fluid drainage from or injection into an area.

Continent urinary diversion

a form of urinary diversion that is able to store urine. The urine is emptied several times a day by placing a catheter into a small channel that connects the conduit to the abdominal wall and allows the urine to drain through the catheter.

Ostomy bag

a specialized bag that is applied over an ostomy to collect urine and stool.

Orthotopic

in the normal or usual position.

Risk

the chance or probability that a particular event will or will not happen.

opening onto the skin is called a **urostomy**. Urine collects in the bag, which is then drained into a toilet several times each day. Second, the bowel can be sewn into a rough sphere connected to the skin by only a small, long channel. This channel prevents urine from leaking out but easily accommodates a small **catheter**. This is called a **continent urinary diversion**. With this type of diversion, you must pass a catheter into the new bladder several times a day to drain the urine. This allows you to live without an **ostomy bag**, but for some patients, passing the catheter several times a day may be difficult or impossible. Third, the new bladder can be directly reattached to the urethra (called an **orthotopic neobladder**). This allows you to urinate almost normally, although you do need to learn to use different muscles, as the new bladder replacement is not able to contract on its own. This is an excellent option for some people, but it is a longer, more difficult operation with some **risk** of **incontinence**. For more details on these procedures and more discussion about which option may be right for you, see Question 80.

3. What is cancer?

To understand **cancer**, we must first understand normal functioning of the body. The body is made up of billions of **cells**. Each **organ** of the body is made up of several different types of specialized cells. For example, the liver has cells that filter toxins from the blood, and the brain has **nerve** cells (called neurons) that are able to conduct electrical signals. Perhaps the most familiar cells are skin cells. Every flake of dry skin is made of millions of cells that are constantly dying and being replaced with new cells. The growth of new cells is carefully balanced to occur at the same rate as the death of old cells. Your body has many mechanisms in place to regulate the timing of the birth and death of cells. Unfortunately, if one of these mechanisms malfunctions, the careful balance can be disrupted. Environmental toxins such as cigarette smoke, chemicals, and **radiation** can damage **DNA** and can disrupt these control mechanisms. A **tumor** may develop when new cells are created faster than old cells die. Tumors can be either **benign** or **malignant**. A benign tumor is an overgrowth of cells that is unchecked by the body's normal mechanisms; thus, it will keep getting bigger. It is called benign because it does not cause you illness. Some benign tumors can get to be so large that they do cause problems, especially if they are in a confined space, such as your skull. A malignant tumor is also an overgrowth of cells. The tumor is considered malignant, however, because the cells are no longer confined to the tumor. Cells may spread from the main tumor through the blood and **lymph system** or grow directly into nearby structures. As the cells begin to grow unchecked in new organs, they gradually cause dysfunction all over the body and may eventually even cause death.

4. What is bladder cancer?

Bladder cancer is a malignant overgrowth of the cells of the bladder. Most commonly, the growth occurs in cells that are in the urothelium. The lining of most hollow spaces in the body is made of **epithelial cells**. The lining of the inside of your cheek, for instance, is

Incontinence
the involuntary loss of urine.

Cancer
abnormal and uncontrolled growth of cells in the body that may spread, injure areas of the body, and lead to death.

Cell
the smallest unit of the body. Tissues in the body are made of cells.

Organ
tissues in the body (i.e., heart, bladder) that work together to perform a specific function.

Nerve
a cord-like structure composed of a collection of nerve fibers that conveys impulses between a part of the central nervous system and some other region of the body.

Radiation
the application of energy in the form of rays or waves to treat various medical conditions.

The Basics

DNA

the basic building block of cells. It carries the cells genetic information and hereditary characteristics.

Tumor

an abnormal swelling or mass.

Benign

a noncancerous tumor that can expand and press on surrounding structures but does not invade surrounding structures and does not spread to a distant site.

Malignant

a cancerous tumor; can invade surrounding structures and spread to a distant site.

Lymphatic system

the tissues and organs (the bone marrow, spleen, thymus, and lymph nodes) that produce and store cells that fight infection and the network of vessels that carry lymph.

Epithelial cells

cells that cover the surface of the body and line its cavities.

an epithelial cell lining. Also, the lining of your stomach, bowels, **gallbladder** and—you guessed it, the bladder—is made of epithelial cells. Each organ has its own subset of epithelial cells. In the bladder, the lining cells are called transitional epithelial cells. The cancer that grows from these cells is then called **transitional cell cancer**; 90% to 95% of all bladder cancers are of this type. If the cancer grows from a different type of cell in the bladder, it is given a different name. Other types of uncommon cancers in the bladder include **squamous cell carcinoma** and **adenocarcinoma** (**carcinoma** is another word for cancer). A very rare type of bladder cancer that only occurs in children is called **rhabdomyosarcoma**.

It is also possible that cancer in the bladder did not begin there but spread to the bladder from somewhere else. The bladder is an uncommon place for other tumors to "seed" (or **metastasize**), but it does occasionally occur. Although metastases are uncommon, tumors can occasionally grow directly into the bladder from an adjacent organ, such as the prostate, colon, rectum, or **cervix**.

5. How common is bladder cancer?

Cancer is one of the major causes of death and **disease** throughout the world. If all types of cancer are combined, it ranks as the second leading cause of death in the United States today behind heart disease. As treatments for heart disease continue to improve, it has been estimated that within the next 5 to 10 years cancer will become the leading cause of death in the United States and other developed countries.

Bladder cancer is the fourth most common type of cancer in men and the eighth most common in women. Overall, it accounts for approximately 10% of all cancers in men and 4% of all cancers in women. In 2002, it was estimated that 56,500 new bladder cancers were diagnosed in the United States and that there were 12,600 bladder cancer-related deaths. In the last 10 years, the annual number of new cases of bladder cancer has increased by 36%; the good news, however, is that the number of deaths each year from bladder cancer has decreased during that same time by 8%. This is largely because of improved detection of early bladder cancer and improved treatments for advanced bladder cancer.

Bladder cancer is more than 2.5 times more common in men than in women. It is estimated that a white male born in 1997 has a 3.7% chance of developing bladder cancer at some point in his life. The **incidence** of bladder cancer increases with age in both sexes, meaning that an older individual is more likely to acquire bladder cancer than a younger person. It is twice as common in white American men as it is in African American men and 1.5 times more common in white American women as it is in African American women. Hispanic Americans also have about half the rates of bladder cancer as do white Americans. Bladder cancer is more common in the United States and Great Britain than in Japan or Finland.

Although bladder cancer is more common in white Americans, African Americans tend to have more advanced disease when they first present to the doctor. This may be because of an underreporting of more **superficial** tumors, delays in **diagnosis**, or a tendency toward more aggressive tumors in this group. As would

The Basics

Gallbladder

a digestive tract organ that stores bile, a chemical produced in the liver.

Squamous cell carcinoma

of the bladder, a type of cancer that typically occurs in chronically inflamed bladders, such as occurs in individuals with chronic indwelling catheters.

Adenocarcinoma

a form of cancer that develops from a malignant abnormality in the cells lining a glandular organ; a less common form of cancer of the bladder.

Carcinoma

a form of cancer that originates in tissues that line or cover a particular organ.

Rhabdomyo-sarcoma

a malignant tumor derived from striated skeletal muscle.

Metastasize

describes when a cancerous tumor has spread to a distant site, for example, the bones, the liver, or the brain.

Cervix

the lower and narrow end of the uterus, connects to the vagina.

Disease

any change from or interruption of the normal structure or function of any part or organ system of the body that presents with characteristic symptoms and signs, whose cause and prognosis may be known or unknown.

Incidence

the rate at which a certain event occurs, for example, the number of new cases of a specific disease occurring during a certain period.

Superficial

near the surface.

Diagnosis

the identification of the cause or presence of a medical problem or disease.

Papillary

related to bladder cancer, a bladder cancer that has a stalk with nipple-like projections.

Sessile

pertaining to bladder cancer, a cancer that is broad based, stalkless.

be expected from the tendency toward more advanced disease, 5-year survival rates are 71% for African American men versus 84% for white men, and 71% for African American women versus 76% for white women.

6. Are there different types of bladder cancer?

Yes. There are two broad types of cancers in the bladder: primary and metastatic. Primary bladder cancers are those that begin in the bladder itself. Metastatic cancers are those that originated in another organ and then spread to the bladder. Other tumors can get into the bladder through the bloodstream, through the lymphatic system, or by directly extending from a nearby organ, such as the prostate or the cervix.

Primary bladder cancers are far more common than metastatic bladder cancers. There are several types of primary tumors. Recall that transitional cell cancer accounts for at least 90% of all bladder cancers. Transitional cell tumors can be (1) **papillary**, looking like a cauliflower attached to the wall by a short stalk; (2) **sessile**, looking flat and broad-based; or (3) a mix of both. Almost 70% of transitional cell tumors are papillary types, which tend to have a better **prognosis** than sessile tumors. Less common types of bladder cancer include squamous cell cancer, adenocarcinoma, and **urachal carcinoma** (Figure 2).

Squamous cell carcinoma accounts for 3% to 7% of bladder cancers in the United States. In Egypt, it accounts for 75% of the bladder cancers. There is a parasitic infection called **schistosomiasis** that is very common in Egypt. Infection with this **parasite**

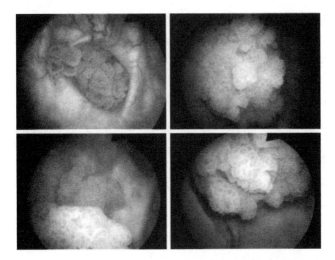

Figure 2   Papillary transitional cell carcinoma of the bladder. Reprinted with permission © Healthcommunities.com Inc., 2005. All rights reserved.

strongly predisposes a person to the development of squamous cell cancer. It is thought that the infection sets up a chronic irritation in the bladder that over many years leads to the development of this type of cancer. Other conditions that cause chronic irritation also predispose to this type of tumor. Chronic indwelling catheters, for example, can irritate the bladder and predispose someone to this tumor. Squamous cell carcinoma does not tend to spread to the **lymph nodes** like transitional cell cancer does, although it does tend to spread aggressively directly through the bladder into neighboring structures. Because it is so locally aggressive and relatively resistant to **chemotherapy** or radiation, it usually has a worse prognosis than transitional cell cancers.

Prognosis

the long-term outlook or prospect for survival and recovery from a disease.

Urachal carcinoma

cancer that develops in the urachus. Although classified as a bladder cancer, this cancer develops outside of the bladder and grows into the bladder.

Schistosomiasis

a parasite that is a "fluke" or "worm."

Parasite

an organism that obtains food and shelter from another organism.

11

Lymph nodes

a small bean-shaped organ that is part of the immune system; nodes filter out bacteria or cancer cells that may travel though the lymphatic system.

Chemotherapy

a treatment for cancer that uses powerful medications to weaken and to destroy the cancer cells.

Adenocarcinoma of the bladder is quite uncommon, accounting for approximately 2% of all bladder cancers in the United States. These tumors are also associated with chronic irritation. They tend to be high-grade aggressive tumors and are therefore usually associated with a worse prognosis.

Urachal carcinoma is a specific type of adenocarcinoma of the bladder, but it is unique in that it does not originate in the lining of the bladder. These develop from the outer surface of the bladder, extending toward the inside of the bladder. They can then metastasize to the lymph nodes, the liver, lung, and bone.

7. What causes bladder cancer?

Cancer, including bladder cancer, develops because of changes in the DNA of a normal cell. DNA can be damaged by chemical exposures such as cigarette smoke, industrial chemicals, chemotherapy, and so forth. (See Questions 10 and 11.) Environmental exposures such as these are called risk factors. Risk factors do not exactly *cause* bladder cancer. Not everyone who smokes will get bladder cancer. However, as a group, the risk is elevated relative to people who do not smoke. Exposures such as these increase the likelihood of DNA becoming damaged. When the specific DNA that controls a cell's growth is damaged, the cell then has the potential to become cancerous. The hallmark of cancer is overgrowth of cells, causing compression of surrounding **tissues** or destruction of the tissues.

Tissue

specific type of material in the body, such as muscle, hair.

8. Can I do anything to avoid getting bladder cancer?

Absolutely! Some risk factors, such as your **genes**, cannot be changed. Many more, however, can be changed. Cigarette smoking is the biggest risk factor for getting bladder cancer. If you are a smoker, the most important thing you can do is to quit today. If someone you live with smokes, encourage that person to quit also. Question 10 discusses what are called modifiable risk factors. These are the **lifestyle** and environmental things that you can change to decrease your chances of getting bladder cancer. Look over this list carefully, and do everything you can to change your lifestyle now to help protect your future and your family's future.

Genes

located in the nucleus of the cell, genes contain hereditary information that is transferred from cell to cell.

Lifestyle

the way a person chooses to live.

9. What are my risk factors for bladder cancer that I cannot change (unmodifiable risk factors)?

As we alluded to previously here, not everyone has the same risk of developing cancer. By studying the characteristics of patients who have bladder cancer, researchers have been able to identify groups of people who seem to develop the disease more often than others. These groups of people each have some risk factor that they are born with, things that predispose them to cancer no matter how carefully they live their lives. In fact, our genetic makeup probably plays the biggest role in determining who among us is destined to get cancer.

Race: Different races have different risks of bladder cancer. Caucasian (white) Americans are twice as likely to develop transition cell cancer (the most common

The Basics

type of bladder cancer), as are African Americans. For the more rare type of bladder cancer, called squamous cell cancer, however, the reverse is true; African Americans are twice as likely to develop squamous cell cancer of the bladder than are white individuals. Of all the different races, Caucasians seem to have the highest rate of bladder cancer.

Gender: Men are almost three times more likely to develop cancer than women. This is before taking into consideration modifiable risk factors such as smoking and workplace exposures to chemicals.

Age: More than 65% of bladder cancer occurs in patients who are older than 65. Patients in this age group are also more likely to develop more aggressive tumor types than are the younger bladder cancer patients.

Genetics: As you may remember from the prior discussion, cancer develops only after something goes haywire in the regulatory process of cell growth or cell death. Several different genes normally accomplish this regulation. In a normal, healthy cell, these genes promote growth or suppress growth or can even signal a cell to destroy itself in an appropriate situation. For a cell to become cancerous, many of these genes must be altered or destroyed simultaneously. Nature has even supplied our cells with other genes that are able to repair damaged genes. These "repairmen" genes are known as **tumor suppressor genes**. Their job is to repair damaged DNA when possible or to drive a damaged cell to destroy itself.

The net result of these processes is to strike a balance of new cell growth and old cell death. You can imagine

Tumor suppressor genes

a group of genes that act to slow down the growth/ development of a cancer/tumor.

that if there were damage to the process that removes cells, then these cells would begin to accumulate. If many other cells also were missing this signal, they might all live too long, causing an overgrowth of cells that we refer to as a tumor. If the cells simply accumulate, then we call the tumor benign. If the cells are able to escape from the main tumor and begin to accumulate in other organs, we refer to the tumor as malignant.

Fortunately, nature is not so easily beaten, and there are multiple redundant systems to regulate these cell cycles. For cancer to develop, there needs to be damage to multiple systems at the same time. When cancer runs in a family, it is usually because damage to one or more of these systems is present already, making it much easier to have a failure of regulation later in life. Examples of these genes are the p53 gene or the retinoblastoma (Rb) gene. Damage to p53 is the most common genetic change in all types of cancers.

Although these systems normally provide tight regulation of cell growth, your body does not *always* want tight regulation. Sometimes cells need to be able to reproduce quickly without the constraints of the regulatory genes. Examples of this include the healing phase after an injury or surgery, or during normal growth in childhood. To accommodate these situations, there are other genes in each cell that when activated allow the cell to grow more vigorously. When you break a bone, new bone cells need to move in quickly and replace the damaged tissue. Your body then needs a way "take off the brakes" to allow growth of certain cell types. A common signal to "hit the accelerator" is called **epidermal growth factor** and is often abnormal in bladder cancer, especially in more aggressive tumors. These types of genes are known as

Epidermal growth factor

a chemical that stimulates growth of cells.

100 QUESTIONS & ANSWERS ABOUT BLADDER CANCER

Oncogenes

genes that can potentially induce neoplastic transformation (development of cancer).

P21 ras oncogene

a specialized oncogene that has been associated with cancers in humans.

Proteins

any group of complex organic macromolecules that contain carbon, hydrogen, oxygen, nitrogen, and usually sulfur and are composed of alpha-amino acids. Proteins are fundamental components of all living cells and include many substances such as enzymes, hormones, and antibodies that are necessary to the functioning of an organism.

Aniline dyes

a class of synthetic, organic dyes obtained from aniline (coal tars). These dyes have been used to impart color to paper, cloth, and leather, and have been used in woodworking.

oncogenes. A gene named the **p21 ras oncogene** can be found in many bladder cancers. Although oncogenes are not well understood, they may play a role in determining how aggressively a tumor behaves. They appear able to change a low-grade tumor into a higher-grade, more aggressive tumor. Researchers are always identifying new genes and new **proteins** that are involved in bladder cancer, and each new finding provides a possible route of new therapy to prevent or treat bladder cancer.

10. What are the risk factors for bladder cancer that I could change?

There are several known risk factors for bladder cancer. By far the biggest cause of bladder cancer in the United States is cigarette smoking. Other risk factors are exposure to **aniline dyes**, recurrent **urinary tract infections**, chronic **foley catheters**, bladder stones, and previous radiation to the pelvis as treatment for another cancer. Also, there may be a small increased risk for people who color their hair with permanent hair colors, with the risk increased in those people who dye their hair more often or who started coloring it at a younger age. Dietary factors may also affect the risk of bladder cancer. In a review of data from the Surveillance, Epidemiology, and End Results database, it was found that patients with other primary tumors had a tenfold higher risk of bladder cancer compared with the general population. The risk was highest in patients who were previously diagnosed with prostate cancer. Infection of the bladder by a parasite called schistosomiasis markedly increases the risk of bladder cancer. Although this infection is common in Egypt and surrounding countries, it is rare in the United States.

Tobacco: Cigarette smoking accounts for 25% to 65% of all cases of bladder cancer in the United States. It increases the risk of bladder cancer by up to four times compared with someone who has never smoked. As you might expect, the risk increases as the number of cigarettes increases, the number of years of smoking increases, and by the degree of inhalation with each puff. This applies to both men and women. The risk is even higher with the use of air-cured "black" tobacco because it has a higher concentration of chemicals than flue-cured "blond" tobacco. The good news is that quitting smoking decreases your risk; thus, it is never too late to quit. Other forms of tobacco, such as cigars and smokeless tobacco, also increase the risk of cancer, although to a lesser degree. It is not clear what chemical in the cigarette smoke is responsible for bladder cancer. Some people clear the chemicals from cigarette smoke more slowly than others do. These people, called **slow acetylators**, appear to be at increased risk for bladder cancer.

Occupational risk factors: Exposure to aniline dyes is the most common industrial risk factor for bladder cancer. Aniline dyes are byproducts of burning coal. These dyes have been used for staining or coloring wood and textiles. Other occupational chemicals that have also been associated with bladder cancer include 2-naphthylamine, 4-aminobiphenyl, 4-nitrobiphenyl, 4-4-diaminobiphenyl (benzidine), and 2-amino-1-naphthol, certain aldehydes used in rubber and textile manufacturing, combustion gases and soot from coal, and possibly hydrocarbons. An increased risk has been reported in all of the following occupations: autoworker, painter, truck driver, drill press operator, leather worker, metal worker, machine operator, dry

Urinary tract infection

infection of the urinary tract with microorganisms. It may involve the bladder (cystitis) and/or the kidney (pyelonephritis).

Foley catheter

a catheter that is placed into the bladder via the urethra to drain urine.

Slow acetylator

someone who metabolizes certain chemicals more slowly.

The Basics

cleaner, paper manufacturer, rope and twine maker, dental technician, barber, hairdresser, physician, apparel manufacturer, and plumber.

Phenacetin: Phenacetin is a pain medication that is no longer available in this country, although it is still available in other countries. Large doses have been shown to increase the likelihood of developing bladder cancer.

Pelvic radiation: Pelvic radiation increases the risk of developing bladder cancer. Women who have undergone **radiation therapy** for uterine cancer or ovarian cancer in the past now have a twofold to fourfold higher risk of developing bladder cancer. The risk of bladder cancer increases even more if chemotherapy was combined with the radiation. Similarly, men who have had radiation therapy for prostate cancer also have an elevated risk of bladder cancer.

Radiation therapy

the use of high-energy radiation to destroy cancer cells; also called radiotherapy or irradiation.

Chemotherapy and immunosuppression: Chemotherapy with the drug cyclophosphamide is associated with up to a ninefold increased risk of developing bladder cancer. These cancers tend to be more aggressive as a group. Also, patients who have had a kidney transplant or other organ transplants and are on immunosuppression (steroids and other medications) are known to have a higher risk for bladder cancer.

Dehydration: Individuals who typically take in very little fluids are at increased risk of developing bladder cancer. Minimizing fluid intake causes the urine to become more concentrated and increases the amount of time between voiding. Holding concentrated urine for longer periods of time likely plays a role in this increased risk.

11. Are there dietary changes I could make that can reduce my risk of bladder cancer?

The risk of developing bladder cancer appears to correlate with fat and cholesterol intake. Some studies have suggested that eating a low-fat, low-cholesterol diet may decrease your risk of developing cancer.

A recent study from Japan showed a decreased risk of bladder cancer in patients who had diets that were high in green vegetables or carrots. Those who ate five or more servings per week were half as likely to develop bladder cancer, as were those who ate one to three servings per month.

Soy protein and garlic intake may also decrease the risk. Garlic has been shown to have a direct toxic effect on bladder cancer cells grown in a culture dish in the laboratory. This effect may be due to stimulating the body's natural defenses to kill cancerous cells.

Some vitamins have also been found to have anticancer effects, although little information is specifically related to their effects on bladder cancer (Table 1).

In a recent study of almost a million adults, those who were cigarette smokers and regularly took vitamin E for 10 years or longer had a decreased risk of death from bladder cancer. The effect was less in nonsmokers. Smokers who took vitamin E were, however, still at **high risk** for bladder cancer; thus, avoiding cigarettes is still important! There was no decreased risk in those who took vitamin C.

The Basics

High risk
more likely to have a complication or side effect.

Table 1   Vitamins with Potential Anticancer Effects

Vitamin	Food Source	Effects
E	Wheat germ, cereals, nuts, spinach, egg yolk	Antioxidant; Prevents the production of toxic metabolites such as nitrosamines
C	Citrus fruit, black currants, potatoes, tomatoes, green chilies	Antioxidant and free-radical scavenger
B6	Cabbage	Corrects abnormal tryptophan metabolism found in 50% of bladder cancer patients
A	Animal products and green and yellow vegetables	May decrease risk of developing some cancers

If you are confused about all of the different recommendations for a "healthy" diet, you are not alone. It is difficult to study the effects of diet on any disease because it requires hundreds or thousands of patients making strict changes to their diet for many years. Anyone who has ever tried a new diet can imagine how difficult it is to find volunteers who are reliably able to do this! The best recommendation, therefore, is to use common sense and to be wary of any expensive pills that claim to be highly effective. Eat a balanced diet with fruit, meat, breads, and vegetables without overdoing any one item. Quit smoking, and exercise regularly. Even without a scientific study, we can all agree that those three things will keep you healthy.

12. Does everyone have the same chance of developing bladder cancer?

The overall chance of developing bladder cancer during your lifetime is 3% to 4%. This type of number, however, lumps the entire world into one group.

In order to create a more meaningful number, researchers try to identify who is at a higher or lower risk. Factors in the environment or one's lifestyle that increase the risk of developing cancer are called risk factors.

There are two types of risk factors. Risk factors that we are born with, such as our family **genetics** or race, are called *unmodifiable risk factors* because we cannot change them. For example, a man is two and a half times more likely to develop bladder cancer than is a woman, and there is no way for him to decrease this risk.

The second type of risk factor is called a *modifiable risk factor*. You can change these risk factors to decrease your odds of developing cancer. The most obvious modifiable risk factor is tobacco. Smoking dramatically increases your risk of developing cancer, and quitting smoking dramatically decreases that risk. The next two questions discuss these risks in more detail.

13. A family member of mine has bladder cancer. Am I at high risk?

No strong evidence at present suggests that bladder cancer may be passed from parent to child. There have been reports of families with several members who have bladder cancer, but these did not take into account risk factors such as cigarette smoking or exposure to environmental toxins. Family members tend to be exposed to similar toxins, and thus it is difficult to make conclusions from these studies. It clear is that most people with bladder cancer do not have a strong family **history** of bladder cancer.

Genetics

a field of medicine that studies heredity.

History

an oral or written interview that consists of questions about your medical, social, and family background.

The Basics

14. I have bladder cancer. Is my family at risk?

Bladder cancer is *not* contagious. It cannot be transmitted from person to person. You cannot spread it to your family or friends, and they cannot catch it from you. As we just mentioned, however, family members do tend to be exposed to similar toxins, such as cigarette smoke and environmental chemicals; thus, they may have an increased risk of developing cancer from these other sources.

15. Is there a cure for bladder cancer?

When we refer to someone as being "cured" of a disease, we generally mean that the disease is gone forever and will not recur. When we refer to a person's cancer as cured, we generally refer to a period that must elapse with no evidence of **recurrence**.

Recurrence

the reappearance of disease.

For many patients, there is indeed a cure for bladder cancer. Those patients with low-grade, superficial cancer will in a sense be cured when they undergo removal of their entire tumor. Unfortunately, bladder cancer tends to recur in other areas of the bladder. Even though the entire tumor was removed, new tumors can grow in either the same or different locations. Thus, despite having had your entire tumor removed, you will still need to be monitored regularly. Many recurrent tumors, when detected early, are still curable tumors.

For those patients with tumors that have invaded the bladder muscle, cure is still possible. Either part or all of the bladder can be removed. If the surgeon is able to remove the entire tumor, then you are said to be cured of the cancer. Surgery will cure approximately 80% of the tumors that are confined to a person's bladder. Unfortunately, again, it is impossible to know for certain that the entire tumor has been removed. **Microscopic** amounts of tumor may have escaped the bladder, and the surgeon has no way of detecting when this happens. In cases in which this is suspected, such as the presence of tumor cells at the edge of the removed tissue, chemotherapy or radiation may be added to improve the chances of curing the microscopic tumor that remains in the body. Patients with **locally advanced** cancer have only about a 20% to 30% chance of cure with surgery alone. Surveillance by a **urologist** after surgery is always important to ensure that the tumor does not recur.

Finally, those patients who develop metastatic cancer can still be cured. Combination therapy with surgery, chemotherapy, and/or radiation is now able to cure a small but growing number of these patients. Most patients will at least respond initially to chemotherapy. As with the other examples, it is difficult to say at what point we can call a patient cured. Surveillance with X-rays, computerized tomography (**CT**) **scans**, **cystoscopy**, and **cytology** remains important for years after therapy.

16. What is carcinoma in situ?

Carcinoma in situ of the bladder is a type of cancer. Carcinoma in situ in other parts of the body, such as the prostate, cervix, or **testicle**, is thought to be a **premalignant** condition, but in the bladder it is always malignant. If untreated, 50% of cases will progress to muscle-invasive cancer within 5 years, and thus carcinoma in situ needs to be taken very seriously. The rate

Locally advanced
describes when a cancerous tumor has spread to surrounding structures.

Urologist
a doctor who specializes in the evaluation and treatment of diseases of the genitourinary tract in males and females.

CT scan
a specialized X-ray study that allows one to visualize internal structures in cross-section to look for abnormalities.

Cystoscopy
the procedure of using a cystoscope to look into the urethra and bladder.

Cytology
the study of cells under a microscope.

Carcinoma in situ
pertaining to bladder cancer, a superficial-appearing bladder cancer that is associated with a high risk of subsequent invasive disease.

Testicle
the male reproductive organ that produces testosterone and sperm. Normally, there are two that are located in the scrotum.

The Basics

of **progression** to **invasive** cancer is even worse for those patients who also have a papillary bladder tumor. Carcinoma in situ itself is a flat (not papillary) lesion, and thus it can be more difficult to identify during a cystoscopy. It may appear as a red, irritated patch or may be indistinguishable from normal, adjacent bladder. If a patient is at high risk for carcinoma in situ, most urologists will take random biopsies of the bladder to screen for this disease even though the bladder may appear normal at the time of the cystoscopy. Carcinoma in situ tends to shed cells into the urine, which can usually be detected on a urine sample by a test called **urine cytology** (see Question 33 for more details).

17. What is dysplasia?

Dysplasia is thought to be the precursor to carcinoma in situ and/or invasive bladder cancer. Dysplasia refers to the appearance of cells under the microscope. They do not appear normal, but they also do not have the usual hallmarks of cancer. It is, however, frequently found in patients who have either carcinoma in situ or bladder cancer. More than 50% of patients with bladder cancer have dysplasia. It is more common in men than women. Although dysplasia is not actually cancer or even precancer, it is thought to be a marker for an "unstable" urothelium, which may go on to develop cancer. Dysplasia does not require any intervention but may be a marker of people who are at risk of developing cancer in the future.

18. Is dysplasia dangerous?

Dysplasia is not well studied, but it is not thought to be dangerous. It represents an in-between category that is neither normal nor cancerous. Approximately one third of patients with pure dysplasia will have **irritative**

voiding symptoms, one third will have **hematuria**, and one third will have no **symptoms** at all. Some patients will have an abnormal urine cytology result. Approximately 20% of patients with dysplasia will eventually develop carcinoma in situ or bladder cancer.

19. What is urachal cancer?

Urachal carcinoma is an uncommon type of bladder cancer. At the M.D. Anderson Cancer Center, one of the largest centers in the world, only 42 cases of urachal carcinoma were seen during a 16-year period. It affects men and women equally, although patients are usually younger than most bladder cancer patients. It is a cancer that arises at the dome (top) of the bladder where the **urachal ligament** attaches, connecting the bladder to the umbilicus (navel). It usually is not picked up until it is relatively advanced, making it much harder to treat than more common types of bladder cancer. Twenty percent of patients will have metastases when first identified, and almost all will have tumors invading surrounding organs. Eventually, approximately half of all patients develop metastases.

20. My bladder cancer was successfully treated. Is there anything I can do to keep it from coming back?

The prevention of bladder tumor recurrences is a combined effort between you and your physician. All of the risk factors for getting bladder cancer (Questions 9 and 10) still apply. Quitting smoking is always at the top of the list, as well as avoiding other carcinogens on the list, such as aniline dyes. In addition to these preventative measures, your physician might recommend treatments that are designed to reduce the likelihood that

Irritative voiding symptoms

the symptoms of urinary frequency and urgency.

Hematuria

the presence of blood in the urine. It may be gross (visible) or microscopic (only detected under the microscope).

Symptom

subjective evidence of a disease, that is, something that the patient describes, such as pain in the abdomen.

Urachal ligament

the remnant of the urachus.

The Basics

BCG

as it pertains to bladder cancer, live attenuated tuberculosis bacteria that are placed into the bladder (intravesical therapy) to decrease the recurrence of bladder cancer.

Interferon

a substance produced by cells that suppresses the growth of cells and regulates the immune response.

Mitomycin C

a chemical that prevents the production of DNA and that prevents cell growth.

Thiotepa

a form of chemotherapy used intravesically for bladder cancer.

the cancer will recur. These include but are not limited to immune therapy with **BCG** (*Bacillus Calmette-Guerin*; see Question 52) or **interferon** (see Question 57), chemotherapy with **mitomycin C, thiotepa,** and other agents. These agents are placed directly into the bladder to kill cancer cells (Question 49). Ask your doctor whether any of these treatments might help to reduce your risk of experiencing a recurrence.

PART TWO

Diagnosis

What are the signs and symptoms of bladder cancer?

Are there other conditions that can cause hematuria?

My doctors suspect I have bladder cancer.
What tests will I need?

More . . .

21. What are the signs and symptoms of bladder cancer?

One of the most common **signs** of bladder cancer is blood in the urine (hematuria). In the majority of cases, this includes microscopic amounts of blood that can only be picked up by the laboratory on a urine sample. Some people will have so much bleeding that it turns the urine pink or red (gross hematuria). Obviously, gross hematuria is not normal, and because it is so alarming, it will often prompt quicker evaluation. Microscopic hematuria though is also not normal and should always be evaluated by a urologist. Even if the blood in the urine clears up on its own, it still always needs to be evaluated. The absence of pain does not mean that there is no need for concern.

Hematuria is not the only warning sign, however. Depending on its location within the bladder, the tumor may interfere with the normal functioning of the bladder, which could manifest as irritative voiding symptoms. These symptoms include urinary urgency and urinary **frequency**. Urgency is the feeling of a sudden, compelling desire to urinate that is difficult to make go away. Frequency means going to the bathroom eight or more times per day. Urgency and frequency are often caused by a simple urinary tract infection. Kidney stones can also cause these symptoms as they pass through the last part of the ureters. Irritative voiding symptoms such as urgency and frequency are also the most common symptoms of an **overactive bladder**. Overactive bladder is common in both older men and women. Obviously then, these symptoms do not necessarily mean that you have cancer and are not in and of themselves reason to suspect cancer.

Sign

objective evidence of a disease or condition; that is, something the doctor identifies.

Frequency

the need to urinate often. In adults, it is often used to describe the need to urinate eight or more times per day.

Overactive bladder

a syndrome with symptoms of urgency, frequency, nocturia, and sometimes urge incontinence. It is thought to be related to overactivity of the bladder muscle.

If the tumor is located near the **ureteral orifice** (the opening of the ureter into the bladder), it may block the flow of urine from the kidneys and cause an **obstruction**. Obstruction may often lead to back pain, nausea, and vomiting, especially if it occurs quickly. More gradual obstruction is often asymptomatic. Very rarely, both ureteral orifices may become obstructed, leading to low urine output and kidney failure. If the cancer has spread to an area outside of the bladder, then it could cause swelling of the legs or bone pain. Finally, if the tumor is very large, it could be felt as a mass in the lower abdomen.

I was very young when I was diagnosed with bladder cancer. In fact, because I was so young no one even thought that I could have bladder cancer. For several months, I had episodes of urinating bloody urine, which were thought to be urinary tract infections. When I told one of my friends about it she recommended that I have it checked out. So I had my primary care doctor refer me to a urologist. The urologist requested my records and told me that I had never had an infection. The urologist told me that it was not uncommon that young women who present with bloody urine are thought to have a urinary tract infection. But he added that the lack of bacteria in my urine should have alerted my primary care doctor and the emergency room doctors that I had seen that something else was going on.

22. Are there other conditions that can cause hematuria?

Gross hematuria (visible blood in the urine) can be caused by several things other than cancer. A simple urinary tract infection, a kidney stone, a bladder stone, chronic irritation in the bladder, many kidney diseases,

Ureteral orifice

the terminal opening of the ureter. Normally it is located in the bladder.

Obstruction

the state or condition of being blocked/clogged.

Diagnosis

29

and other less common conditions all can cause hematuria. Men with large prostates who strain to void may get bleeding because of rupture of small veins in the prostate. Occasionally, long-distance runners can develop hematuria, presumably because of bladder irritation from the repetitive bouncing. Also, patients who have had pelvic radiation to treat other cancers may develop radiation **cystitis**. Radiation cystitis is a benign but troublesome condition because it often causes persistent bleeding in the bladder that can be difficult to fully stop. Although many of these processes are benign and do not require treatment, a urologist needs to evaluate any blood in the urine to rule out the presence of a tumor.

Cystitis

inflammation of the bladder; may be related to a bacterial infection, viral infection, radiation, or other bladder irritants.

Microscopic hematuria can only be seen in the laboratory on a urine sample. It is defined as three or more red blood cells seen per high-power field under the microscope. In the office, many physicians use a urine dipstick to test the urine for blood, but these are overly sensitive. The test may be falsely positive because of menstruation, some antiseptics, recent exercise, dehydration, or the use of a large amount of vitamin C. The dipstick is a strip of paper that is treated with chemicals. Microscopic amounts of blood in the urine react with the chemicals to change their color. Any urine that shows blood on the dipstick test needs to be looked at under the microscope to determine whether blood is really present.

All of the processes mentioned previously here for gross hematuria can also cause microscopic hematuria. In both gross and microscopic hematuria, the first task is to determine *where* the blood is coming from—that is, one kidney, both kidneys, the ureter, the bladder, the prostate, or the urethra (Figure 1). Women may notice blood on the toilet paper and assume that they have hematuria. This can be the case; however, we must first be sure it is not vaginal or uterine bleeding.

In addition to these medical causes of hematuria, several nonmedical things can often be mistaken for hematuria. Eating an inordinately large number of beets can color the urine red. Dehydration can cause the urine to become quite concentrated and dark, giving the impression of hematuria. **Pyridium**, which numbs the urinary tract and is often prescribed during a urinary tract infection, will turn the urine a bright orange.

Pyridium

a medication that acts as a urinary tract anesthetic. It turns the urine an orange color.

23. My doctors suspect I have bladder cancer. What tests will I need?

Most patients who are being evaluated for bladder cancer are referred because of gross or microscopic blood in the urine. Others may have irritative voiding symptoms such as frequency, urgency, or pain. Finally, some may have a positive urine cytology test or a mass detected on a CT scan that was obtained for some other reason, such as back pain.

Several tests and procedures are used in the initial evaluation of bladder cancer. During your initial visit, your doctor will perform a rectal exam (and a pelvic exam for women) to determine whether the tumor is palpable or extending beyond the bladder. Other common tests include (1) urine cytology or other urine screening test (Questions 33–35), (2) X-rays of the kidneys and ureters (Question 33), and (3) cystoscopy to examine the interior of the bladder directly (Question 24). Your doctor will also perform a **biopsy**, often as part of the resection of the tumor in the operating room. The biopsy is sent to the **pathologist**, who looks

Biopsy

the removal of small sample(s) of tissue for examination under the microscope.

Pathologist

a doctor trained in the evaluation of tissues under the microscope to determine the presence/absence of disease.

at it under the microscope to diagnose accurately the type of cancer and the depth of penetration. Any further tests that you might need will depend on the results of the biopsy.

Regardless of the biopsy results, everyone should get an **upper tract study** (Question 31). Upper tract studies are done to make sure that there is no cancer in your kidneys or ureters that cannot be seen during cystoscopy.

You may also need to have tests for your heart such as an electrocardiogram or an echocardiogram, especially if your doctor is planning **anesthesia** for a biopsy or resection in the operating room. If these tests are abnormal, you may need further evaluation by a cardiologist. Also, some people, especially those older than 50 or those who smoke, may need a chest X-ray before having anesthesia.

Finally, for those patients in whom the cancer is suspected to be advanced, a CT scan of the abdomen and pelvis may be obtained. This scan will help to assess whether the cancer has invaded outside of the bladder as well as to determine whether any lymph nodes are enlarged.

24. What is cystoscopy?

Cystoscopy refers to the direct visual examination of the inside of the bladder using a small telescope called a **cystoscope** (Figure 3). The cystoscope has a light at the tip to illuminate the bladder. There is a channel through which water flows and fills the bladder, stretching it out to allow better visualization. The cystoscope is inserted directly through the urethra so that it can also be seen. You may occasionally see cystoscopy called cysto-urethroscopy, but these are the same thing.

Upper tract study

a radiologic study used to evaluate the kidneys and ureters.

Anesthesia

the loss of feeling or sensation; with respect to surgery, means the loss of sensation of pain, as it is induced to allow surgery or other painful procedures to be performed. General anesthesia is a state of unconsciousness, produced by anesthetic agents, with absence of pain sensation over the entire body and a greater or lesser degree of muscle relaxation. Local anesthesia is confined to one part of the body. Spinal anesthesia is produced by injection of a local anesthetic into the subarachnoid space around the spinal cord.

Cystoscope

a telescope-like instrument that allows examination of the urethra and the inside of the bladder.

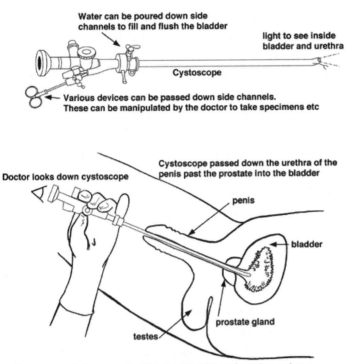

Cystoscopy is the examination the bladder and urethra using a cystoscope (a thin 'telescope')

Figure 3 Cystoscope. This instrument is used to examine the bladder for bladder cancer. Reprinted by permission of Dr. Tom Kenney, author and copyright holder of PILS.

A number of specialized instruments have been created that are able to be passed through the cystoscope. These instruments allow your urologist to take biopsies, inject dyes, crush bladder stones, and use **cautery** inside the bladder. Before the invention of cystoscopy, these procedures would all have required making an **incision** in the abdomen and performing surgery.

A flexible cystoscope is a smaller scope that can be easily used in the office for diagnosis and follow-up. It does not require any anesthesia but has a limited ability to take biopsies, cauterize, and so forth. Often a patient will have a flexible cystoscopy in the office and

Cautery

the application of a caustic substance— a hot instrument, an electric current, or other agent—to destroy tissue or control bleeding.

Incision

cutting of the skin at the beginning of surgery.

33

then go to the operating room only if necessary for biopsy, resection, or **retrograde pyelograms**.

There is little risk to the patient from a simple cystoscopy. After the procedure, you may notice some burning the first couple of times that you urinate after the test. Occasionally, some faint blood will be in the urine. If the burning or irritation persists beyond this, you should contact your doctor, as it could be the sign of a urinary tract infection. To help prevent this, many physicians will prescribe an antibiotic to be taken at the time of the procedure.

When I first saw the cystoscope, I said to my doctor that there was no way that he was putting that instrument where he said he was putting it. It looked like a garden hose to me. But of course, he eventually persuaded me that he needed to do the procedure and that it was best to do it in the office. He told me he would put some numbing jelly into my urethra, and that since the instrument was flexible it would follow the curves and that it was smaller than the opening that I urinated through. Well I didn't think so, but I finally gave in. To tell you the truth, it wasn't half as bad as I envisioned. Now I have the procedure performed every 3 months, and I don't even think twice about it. (N. B., 58 years old)

25. Why do I need a pelvic exam?

A pelvic exam is an important part of evaluating bladder cancer, and all women should have a proper pelvic exam during the initial visit. The pelvic exam helps to determine the **stage** of the tumor. Your doctor places one hand on your abdomen and the other into the vagina during the exam. This enables him or her to feel the bladder, and he or she can often determine whether the tumor has invaded through the wall of the bladder. The pelvic exam also allows evaluation of the uterus and ovaries. Some cancers in the bladder are actually extensions of cervical cancer, uterine cancer, or ovarian cancer and would therefore be treated differently than transitional cell cancer. Most urologists will refer you to a gynecologist if there are any abnormalities found on the pelvic exam.

26. If bladder lesions can be benign or malignant, how do I know which one I have?

An important part of your doctor's evaluation for hematuria is cystoscopy (Question 24), either in the office or in the operating room. Sometimes your doctor can tell just by looking at your bladder wall through the cystoscope that there is a tumor that needs to **resected** in the operating room (Question 38). Other times, there will be an irritated area that could be either benign or malignant. In these cases, a biopsy is necessary to determine the cause of the abnormality. The biopsy is sent to the pathologist who will look at the tissue under the microscope. Under the microscope, it is possible to differentiate between normal bladder cells, cancer cells, **inflammation**, and benign tumors. If the pathologist decides that there is a tumor, he will then assign a **grade** (high or low) to the tumor. If the biopsy is adequate, the pathologist will also report how deep into the wall of the bladder the tumor extends.

Resected

removed surgically.

Inflammation

swelling, redness, pain, and irritation as the result of injury, infection, or surgery.

Grade

with respect to tumors, an assessment of the aggressiveness of the tumor by how the cells look under the microscope.

27. How will the diagnosis of bladder cancer affect me, my spouse/partner, and our relationship?

Each individual is different, and each relationship is different; thus, it is hard to generalize about how each of you and the two of you together will react. In general, there are different aspects of bladder cancer and its treatment that are more stressful for you and your spouse or partner. Men generally are most concerned with the effects of bladder cancer surgery on sexual function and urinary incontinence. Women tend to most concerned with long-term survival. Women with bladder cancer are concerned with the changes in body image that occur, particularly those who have an **ileal conduit**.

Ileal conduit

a form of urinary diversion that uses a piece of small intestine as the conduit.

It appears that as couples face the challenge of dealing with bladder cancer, one of the critical steps is establishing their commitment to each other. This is achieved through communication that may be verbal or nonverbal, such as a hug. The absence of this sense of reconnection between partners, often as a result of failure of communication, can distance the relationship and make mutual support more difficult.

There is a delicate balance for couples between acknowledging fears that arise and keeping them private. Either extreme—being too vocal or too private—appears to create tension. Sometimes men do not express their worries and fears because they are concerned about the effect that this may have on their spouse. They often indicate that they have held things back because they did not want to worry their spouse or felt that their spouses were not strong enough to cope with the issues. It is important that you communicate your concerns and fears with someone—whether it be your physician, close friend or relative, or individuals going through similar experiences—if you feel that you cannot discuss them with your spouse or significant other. You may also ask your physician whether he or she knows of any patients with bladder cancer that are willing to talk about their experience with you and whether there are any bladder cancer support groups in your area.

Confronting a life-threatening illness is difficult, but through open communication and mutual support, it can draw a family closer together, force a reordering of priorities, and influence a change toward a healthier lifestyle for all of those affected.

The day my doctor told me that I had bladder cancer, I went numb. I had to go back to work after my appointment, and I really cannot remember anything that I did that day. All I could do was think about how to break it to my wife. Her father had died of lung cancer, and even though my doctor had told me that my cancer could be treated with therapy that he placed into my bladder and that I would do well, I was really scared to tell her. It took me 2 weeks to tell her the truth. At first I told her that the doctor was still waiting for some test results, but then I finally got up the nerve to tell her the truth. She tried to act like she was sure that I would be fine, but I could tell that she wasn't. She immediately went to the computer and started looking for information on bladder cancer. She had a hard time realizing that the bladder therapy is very different from the chemotherapy that her father received. She came with me to my next appointment and seemed to feel much better after that. She had an opportunity to ask questions, and both of us left the appointment feeling much better. She was very relieved to hear that my urologist did not think that I would ever need chemotherapy like what her father received. (J. S., 68 years old)

28. I am feeling depressed and anxious about my diagnosis of bladder cancer. Is this normal? What can I do to get back to the way I used to be?

The diagnosis of bladder cancer comes as a shock to most individuals. In most individuals, the only symptom/sign of bladder cancer is blood in the urine. Those individuals with gross hematuria (bright red blood in the urine) are usually aware that they need to be evaluated by a physician. Those with microscopic hematuria, however, usually have no real warning that anything is going on. In most cases of bladder cancer, particularly the lower-stage bladder cancers, the individual will feel fine and typically will have no symptoms. Sometimes they will have frequency of urination, but many patients disregard what they interpret as just bothersome symptoms. Thus, when faced with the shock of being diagnosed with bladder cancer, common reactions are fear, anger, confusion, and depression. It is not unusual to retreat initially from life as you absorb the reality of the situation and begin to gather information and start the decision-making process. Many patients will have feelings of failure or guilt, withdraw socially, feel that they are being punished, lose interest in activities that used to bring them pleasure, or find that they are crying a lot. Some will have overwhelming feelings of doom or helplessness and may even think about suicide. These can all be signs of serious depression, and you should discuss this with your doctor immediately. Sometimes, when faced with such potentially overwhelming situations, you may need some assistance to help you gain control of your life again and make the decisions that you will need to make regarding your treatment. Never be afraid to ask for help.

29. What does the tumor grade mean?

Low grade

cancer that does not appear aggressive, advanced.

The pathologist grades a tumor based on how the cells look under the microscope. The tumor cells can appear close to normal (**low grade**) or more aggressive and angry (**high grade**). As you might expect, low-grade tumors tend to have a better prognosis than high-grade tumors. Most pathologists grade tumor biopsies as 1, 2, and 3 instead of high and low. The grade of the tumor allows us to predict who will go on to develop invasive tumors and who will not; 6% of grade I tumors, 52% of grade II tumors, and 82% of grade III tumors will become invasive.

It is harder to define three different grades for a cytology specimen, and thus most urine cytologies are simply reported as high grade or low grade.

30. What are the different stages of bladder cancer?

In addition to determining the grade of the tumor, the pathologist will determine the stage of the tumor (Figure 4), which refers to the extent of the cancer and therefore the chances that it has spread beyond the bladder. The pathologist looks at how deep the tumor invades into the bladder wall. If the cancerous cells are only found in the first layer of the bladder wall (the urothelium), then the cancer is called superficial. If the cells penetrate beyond this into the deeper muscle of the bladder wall, then it is called invasive.

Tumor describes the primary tumor.

- TX: The tumor cannot be assessed.
- T0: No evidence of tumor exists.
- Ta: The tumor is **noninvasive** papillary carcinoma that will not spread.

High grade

very advanced cancer cells.

Diagnosis

Noninvasive

does not extend into the wall of the bladder.

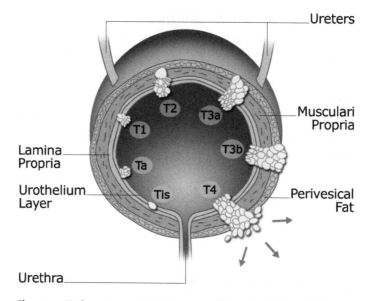

Figure 4 **Various stages of bladder cancer. Illustration by Laura Tritz, reprinted by permission from cancerfacts.com, copyright 2004.**

- Tis: The tumor is confined to the lining of bladder.
- T1: The tumor has spread to the tissue under the bladder lining.
- T2: The tumor has spread to the bladder muscle.
- T3: The tumor has spread to the tissue on the outside of the bladder.
- T4: The tumor has spread to prostate, uterus, vagina, pelvic wall, or abdominal wall.

Nodes describes whether cancer has spread into the lymph nodes in the pelvis.

- NX: The lymph nodes in the pelvis cannot be examined.
- N0: No bladder cancer is found in lymph nodes.

- N1: Bladder cancer is found in one lymph node, 2 cm (0.8 in.) or less in dimension.
- N2: Bladder cancer is found in one or more lymph nodes, none more than 5 cm (2 in.) in dimension.
- N3: Bladder cancer is found in one or more lymph nodes, more than 5 cm (2 in.) in dimension.

Metastasis describes the extent of cancer spread outside of the pelvic region.

Metastasis

the transfer of disease (cancer cells) from one organ or part to another not directly connected with it.

- MX: The spread of cancer to other organs cannot be evaluated.
- M0: No evidence of bladder cancer exists elsewhere in the body.
- M1: Bladder cancer cells are found somewhere else in the body.

Once a tumor's T, N, and M categories have been established, the information is combined in a system called stage grouping that expresses the stage in Roman numerals from I to IV. American Joint Committee on Cancer. (2002). Urinary bladder. In *AJCC Cancer Staging Manual* (6th ed., pp. 335–340). New York: Springer-Verlag.

The stage is very important in determining the treatment that you will receive. There is a good barrier between the urothelium and the muscle of the bladder wall. If the tumor is kept within this barrier, the tumor can usually be completely removed with a **transurethral resection of bladder tumor** (TURBT) (Question 38). If the tumor has become more aggressive, it may figure out how to pass through this barrier. When the tumor has gotten through the protective layer, it becomes much more likely to spread outside of the bladder to

Transurethral resection of bladder tumor (TURBT)

removal of a bladder tumor(s) though a specialized instrument, a resectoscope, that is passed through the penis into the bladder.

other organs or lymph nodes. Once the tumor has gotten through the urothelium, simple scraping of the tumor is not likely to get all of the tumor out, and further therapy will be necessary—either surgery, chemotherapy, or radiation. The option that you and your doctor choose will depend on the extent of spread of the tumor and your overall health status.

Over the years, several different systems have been used to stage cancers. In an effort to ease confusion between different systems, doctors around the world met and decided to create a new **staging** system that would be relevant for all different types of cancer. This system is called **TNM**. The letters stand for *T*umor size, lymph *N*ode status, and the extent of *M*etastases.

It took me about 6 months to finally figure out what this was. All doctor said was, "You have a T2N0 tumor." I'm thinking, "Well, is that good?" I wrote it down on a napkin that I had and kept it in my purse. A few months later, I showed it to my son, who looked it up for me. As it turns out, it is pretty good, as much as any of this is good. (S. R., 68 years old)

31. What are "upper tract studies," and why do I need them?

"Upper tract studies" are evaluations that your doctor does of your kidneys and ureters. The lining of the bladder is the urothelium. The same urothelium also lines the ureters and the inside of the kidneys. The kidneys and the ureters are then also potential locations of transitional cell cancer. The study that your doctor chooses depends on his or her personal opinion

Staging

the process of determining the extent of disease. It is helpful in determining the most appropriate treatment. It often involves physical examination, blood testing, and X-ray studies.

TNM

a specialized cancer staging system that assesses the extent of cancer in the organ the cancer developed in, the lymph nodes, and surrounding/distant tissues/organs.

as well as the availability of each test at your hospital. Even if the upper tract study is **negative**, you will likely need to repeat the studies periodically. Patients with low-grade tumors have a low risk (approximately 2%) of developing upper tract tumors. The presence of a high-grade tumor or of diffuse carcinoma in situ, however, carries up to a 40% lifetime risk of developing an upper tract tumor.

1. An *ultrasound* is often the easiest test to obtain and is therefore popular as a first study. Ultrasound technology generates sound waves and then measures their reflections off of internal structures to produce an image. The same imaging is used for obstetric ultrasounds to produce an image of the fetus. There is no radiation with an ultrasound. An ultrasound is very good for showing tumors and stones in the kidneys and for showing obstruction of the ureter causing **hydronephrosis**. It is not as good for showing small tumors inside the ureter or renal pelvis, and thus a second kind of study is usually needed in addition to the ultrasound.

2. An *intravenous pyelogram* (IVP) is an X-ray study that shows the general outline of the kidneys and better detail of the **collecting system** than an ultrasound. X-ray contrast is given to the patient **intravenously**. The kidneys then filter and concentrate the contrast, creating an image on an X-ray taken a few minutes after the injection is given. A small tumor or stone inside the collecting system can be seen as a dark spot inside the collecting system. An IVP can be performed safely in almost everyone except those people with poorly functioning kidneys or those who have an allergy to intravenous contrast.

Diagnosis

Negative
a test result that does not show what one is looking for.

Ultrasound
a technique used to look at internal organs by measuring reflected sound waves.

Hydronephrosis
dilation of the renal pelvis and calyces of one or both kidneys because of accumulation of urine resulting from obstruction to the outflow of urine.

Intravenous pyelogram
a radiologic study in which a dye is injected into the veins and is picked up by the kidneys and then passed out into the urine. It allows one to visualize the urinary tract.

Collecting system
as it pertains to the kidney, the renal pelvis, and calyces.

Intravenous
into the veins.

3. *CT scanners* use X-rays to create a detailed image of the internal organs. The scanner takes many X-rays at once and uses a computer to combine all of the images into the one picture that you see. When getting a CT scan of the kidneys, the patient is usually scanned twice. The first scan is performed without contrast and will reveal any kidney stones. The second scan is performed with contrast, which helps to show tumors in the kidneys or the collecting system, similar to the IVP but with greater detail. A CT scan is very good for seeing tumors in both the kidneys and the collecting system. In addition to the ability to see the kidneys and ureters better, the CT scan allows for visualization of the entire abdomen and lymph nodes, helping to identify metastases or unrelated diseases. Over the last several years, the cost of CT scans has come down, and the availability of scanners to patients has increased, making the CT scan one of the most common upper tract studies.

As with the IVP test, CT scans meant to examine the kidneys and ureters require intravenous contrast. Patients with kidney disease or allergies to contrast may be better served with a test that does not use contrast, such as a **magnetic resonance imaging** (MRI) or retrograde pyelogram.

Magnetic reso-nance imaging

a study that is similar to a CT scan in that it allows someone to see internal structures in detail, but it does not involve radiation.

4. *MRI* of the kidneys is still a relatively new technology. MRI technology uses magnets to align the molecules in the body. When the magnet is turned off, the molecules revert to their usual state of random directions. As they turn back, they generate a

tiny electrical signal that the MRI machine can detect. These signals are then processed to create a very detailed image. Although an MRI is (in some instances) preferable to a CT scan, it is not generally considered a better test. It is, however, far more costly and often unavailable; thus, it is an uncommon choice for routine upper tract studies. People who have certain surgical implants, such as brain aneurysm clips, cochlear implants, insulin pumps, or other devices, may not be able to have an MRI scan. Also, patients with bullet fragments or shrapnel in their bodies should not have an MRI. The machine itself is similar to a **CT scanner** but can be quite noisy, making it difficult for some people who are claustrophobic. A major advantage of MRI is that it can be performed safely in patients with kidney disease or contrast allergy.

5. *Retrograde pyelograms* are performed by a urologist in the operating room or well-equipped office. While performing cystoscopy, the urologist feeds a catheter into the opening of the ureteral orifice. He or she then injects dye through the catheter, filling the ureter and renal pelvis. An X-ray is obtained that will now show the entire upper tract in good detail. It does not require any intravenous contrast and thus is very useful for patients who are allergic to the contrast or have kidney disease preventing them from receiving contrast. The retrograde pyelogram probably gives the best image of the upper tracts of all of the studies except ureteroscopy. Although the quality of the image is excellent, it does usually require anesthesia and instrumentation that the other studies do not. Therefore, it is most often used in those individuals who are

unable to have one of the previously mentioned X-ray studies or for those patients who have had an abnormality seen on one of those studies.

6. Although *ureteroscopy* is not technically an "upper tract study," it gives us the most definitive examination. It is similar to cystoscopy but uses a smaller scope. In the operating room or well-equipped office, the **ureteroscope** is carefully passed into the ureter as it opens into the bladder. This allows the urologist to see the inside of the ureter. It is gently passed all of the way up the ureter into the kidney. Like cystoscopy, there are both rigid and flexible ureteroscopes. The flexible scope allows doctors to see all or most of the deep corners of the collecting system within the kidney. Biopsies of any suspicious areas can be taken and sent to **pathology** for analysis.

Although ureteroscopy provides the best view of the collecting system, it usually requires anesthesia, and there is some small risk of damage to the kidney or ureter; thus, it is usually reserved for those patients who have had an abnormal upper tract study.

32. What is fluorescence cystoscopy?

Carcinoma in situ can be difficult to see during a routine cystoscopy. Your urologist may take random biopsies of the bladder and send them to pathology, hoping to catch the area that has carcinoma in situ. New technology is available that uses fluorescent lighting through the cystoscope to help identify areas suspicious for carcinoma in situ. A chemical called a **photosensitizer** is instilled into the bladder and is absorbed by the carcinoma in situ cells. When the fluorescent light hits the sensitized cells, they fluoresce, making

Ureteroscope

a long, slender cystoscope-like device that allows one to visualize the ureter, renal pelvis, and calyces.

Pathology

the branch of medicine concerned with disease, especially its structure and functional effects on the body.

Photosensitizer

an agent that makes the tissue photosensitive when applied or absorbed.

them easier to see. This technique is not widely available yet, but can increase detection rates from approximately 70% to 97%.

When this technique was first introduced, the photosensitizer was given intravenously, which had the **side effect** of photosensitizing the skin as well as the tumor. This side effect limited the utility of the treatment. New photosensitizers that are given intravesically are not absorbed systemically, and thus there is no skin **sensitivity** to light, and overall toxicity is minimal.

33. How good is urine cytology?

Urine cytology is commonly used to screen for bladder cancer in patients who have hematuria as well as to monitor for recurrences in patients who are being treated for bladder cancer. Overall, urine cytology is able to detect 40% to 60% of bladder cancers, but the ability of cytology to detect a tumor varies depending on the grade, stage, and location of the tumor. In low-grade, low-stage tumors, cytology will detect 25% to 40% of the tumors. It will perform better as the grade and stage of the tumor increase, with the best detection rate being for carcinoma in situ. Cytology detects approximately 90% of cases of carcinoma in situ. The performance can be improved by sending three separate specimens.

Cytology is less effective when there are other conditions present, such as urinary tract infections, bladder stones, kidney stones, or previous treatment with BCG or intravesical chemotherapy. These conditions all cause inflammation or irritation of the bladder cells, which makes the cytology difficult to interpret.

Side effect
a reaction to a medication or treatment.

Sensitivity
the probability that a diagnostic test can correctly identify the presence of a particular disease.

34. I had a positive urine cytology, but my workup afterward was negative. Do I need to worry?

This is what is usually called a "false-positive" test result. The test was positive in a case where it seems that it should have been negative. Any medical test has a certain false-positive rate (usually very low). The problem with a false-positive result with urine cytology is that there is no way to guarantee the absence of cancer. It is always possible that the cancer is there, but we have not been able to find it yet. Sometimes it can hide in places such as the ureters or kidney where we cannot see as well. Other times, especially with carcinoma in situ, the diseased areas look normal through the cystoscope but actually harbor serious disease. Because of this, one should never ignore a positive cytology result. Close to 80% of patients with a positive cytology but a negative evaluation will eventually be found to have a urologic malignancy.

The current recommendation for patients with a positive urine cytology and a negative initial evaluation is to repeat the urine cytology 6 to 8 weeks later. Those patients with a negative cytology on the follow-up test do not need further evaluation. If the follow-up cytology is positive, however, careful evaluation should be undertaken, as most of these patients will eventually be found to have a malignancy. Your urologist may recommend multiple small biopsies of the bladder to look for carcinoma in situ, a condition that is often associated with positive cytology. Washings may also be obtained from each ureter separately to screen for cancer above the bladder. Finally, you may need to be evaluated for a malignancy in an adjacent organ, such as the colon or uterus, as these tumors can occasionally be the source of an abnormal cytology.

35. Are there tests for bladder cancer other than cytology?

Although cytology has long been the gold standard for bladder cancer screening, including monitoring for recurrences, it is far from perfect (see Question 33), and there is great interest in finding an even better test. Currently, at least four other markers are available, although none of them are clearly better than cytology. In addition to these four, many new tests are being developed. The four listed here are those that are currently available to patients.

NMP 22: **NMP 22** (Matritech, Newton, MA) is a protein that undergoes changes when a bladder cell becomes cancerous. A test for this protein has been developed that looks for the altered protein in the urine; 70% to 80% of patients with bladder cancer will have a positive result, but only 64% of patients with a positive result have cancer. A positive result in a patient without cancer is called a false-positive result. The high false-positive result, often caused by simple inflammation in the bladder, limits its utility.

BTA: **BTA** (Polymedco, Cortlandt Manor, NY) is another protein found in bladder cancer cells but not in normal cells. Tests to detect BTA in the urine are also available. The test identifies 50% to 80% of patients with bladder cancer, but the false-positive rate is similar to NMP 22, limiting its use.

ImmunoCyt: **ImmunoCyt** tests for the presence of three different proteins at the same time. Its ability to detect bladder cancer has varied in different studies from 40% to 100%. The false-positive rate is somewhat better than NMP 22 or BTA at approximately 20%.

Diagnosis

NMP 22

a protein that undergoes changes when a bladder cell becomes cancerous. A urine test has been developed that tests for these changes in NMP 22.

BTA

a protein found in bladder cancer cells but not in normal cells. A urine test is available to check for BTA.

ImmunoCyt

a urine test for bladder cancer. It checks for three different proteins at the same time.

FISH (fluorescent in situ hybridization) (Uro Vysion kit, Visys, Inc./Abbot Laboratories, Downers Grove, IL): This test is able to look directly at the DNA of a cell, searching for malignant cells. Under the microscope, malignant cells light up like a neon sign. It is able to detect more cases of bladder cancer than conventional cytology (73% for **FISH** vs. 63% for cytology) with a false-positive rate of close to 0%. It may detect a tumor up to a year before it can be seen with a cystoscope. Even more, it continues to work well in patients after they have had **intravesical therapy** with BCG or mitomycin C, situations in which cytology does not work well at all. This is an exciting but still new test (approved in 2004), and thus further studies are needed to establish its utility fully in the diagnosis and management of bladder cancer.

36. How do I select a urologist and oncologist?

Once you have been diagnosed with invasive bladder cancer, you should try to select a urologist and **oncologist** who deal with bladder cancer on a regular basis. Several issues should be considered when you select a physician.

Competence: You need a capable doctor who is knowledgeable and can apply that knowledge.

Technical skills: If you are considering a radical **cystectomy**, you want an individual who regularly performs that operation. A radical cystectomy is a complicated, time-consuming procedure that some urologists rarely or never perform. The old dictum "practice makes perfect" certainly applies here. Furthermore, if you are interested in the neobladder option for reconstruction

FISH—fluorescent in situ hybridization

a test that looks directly at the DNA of a cell to identify malignant cells.

Intravesical therapy

medical therapy that is placed into the bladder to kill cancer cells. The therapy is placed into the bladder through a urethral catheter.

Oncologist

a physician who specializes in treating cancer. Urologic oncologists specialize in surgical therapy for cancers of the genitourinary tract. Medical oncologists specialize in treatment with chemotherapy, hormonal therapy, and biologic therapy; and radiation oncologists specialize in treating with radiation.

of your urinary tract, you should make sure that the urologist is comfortable with that portion of the operation. The neobladder adds complexity to the procedure for the surgeon, and not all urologists are well trained in this area. The urologist should know his or her own **complication** rate for the procedure and not just quote widely published rates for other surgeons. He or she should be comfortable and willing to discuss these rates with you.

Compassion: Cancer can be a frightening word and disease no matter how you look at it. You want a physician who understands your fears and concerns and who is willing to take the time to help you make your management decisions. There is no good measure for this, but trust your instincts at your first meeting with a new doctor.

Approachability: As you go through the decision-making process about bladder cancer, you would like your physicians to be available for questions and to be able to answer them in a timely manner. Delays in diagnosis and treatment will add to your anxiety.

My first urologist was just who my doctor told me to go see. He was always running in the room, all out of breath. One day, he just said to me, "You have bladder cancer. The nurse will call you and tell you when to go to the hospital for surgery." Then he made sign a bunch of papers, and that was it. I told my doctor how upset I was, and he found me a young woman urologist who I just love to pieces. She's made it all so much easier for me and my husband. I wish I had gone to her first. (L. R., 66 years old)

Cystectomy

removal of the bladder. Partial cystectomy is removal of a portion of the bladder. Radical cystectomy involves removal of the bladder—in males the prostate and seminal vesicles, and in females the uterus and cervix.

Complication

an undesirable result of a treatment, surgery, or medication.

Diagnosis

37. Do I need to get a second opinion?

Sometimes you may feel that it is necessary to get a second opinion. You may have concerns about the treatment recommendations or may worry that there are other options that have not been presented. If you ever feel that you have not received enough information or that you are uncomfortable with the treatment recommendations from your urologist and/or oncologist, then it is appropriate to seek a second opinion.

Your physicians should be confident enough in their recommendations that they are neither intimidated nor angered by your desire to seek a second opinion. If you experience either of these reactions, then you can be confident in your decision to seek a second opinion. Generally, your physicians will hope that you return to them to discuss the second opinion afterward, especially regarding anything that is divergent from their own recommendations. Most patients return their original caregiver after getting a second opinion, although you are never obligated to do so.

In the end, it is most important that you are comfortable with your treatment plans before beginning therapy. With any form of therapy, it is important to ensure that those physicians at the center where you will be receiving treatment are well experienced with the particular choices that you have made. It is always reasonable to ask your urologist, oncologist, or radiation therapist what his or her (or the institution's) own success rates, failure rates, and complication rates are. If you seek a second opinion, try to compare these rates between the two to help decide which is best suited to you.

As physicians, we often quote the results of large studies published in highly regarded medical journals that show a treatment to be safe and effective. As patients, however, what matters most to you are the results of your local team. If you are concerned because of a lack of information regarding those results, it may be a good time to seek a second opinion.

Some patients are reluctant to seek second opinions because they worry that their doctor will be offended. In reality, any qualified physician understands the difficult decisions that you face and wants you to feel as comfortable as you can with these. In fact, most physicians will help to arrange for copies of your pathology reports, clinic notes, laboratory tests, and X-rays to be sent to the doctor you are seeing for a second opinion. In some areas, your physician will be able to recommend other highly qualified physicians for you to see. It is best if the second physician is not a member of the same group to help ensure objectivity, but when this is your only option, you can rest assured that physicians remain fiercely independent today and will usually give you their honest opinion despite friendships and partnerships.

Diagnosis

53

PART THREE

Treatment

What is a TURBT?

What are the risks of TURBT?

What is perioperative chemotherapy?

More ...

38. What is a TURBT?

TURBT stands for *Trans-Urethral Resection of a Bladder Tumor*. It requires a specialized type of cystoscope that has been modified to include a mechanism to cut out bladder tumors. This specialized scope is called a **resectoscope** and is inserted the same way as a cystoscope. A wire loop is attached that can be extended back and forth (Figure 5).

A small electrical current is passed through the wire loop, giving it the ability to cut through tissue. The loop also cauterizes the tissue, thus preventing bleeding. The loop is then removed, and the cut pieces of tissue are irrigated out of the bladder. The tissue is sent to a pathologist who examines it under a microscope to determine whether it is cancerous. It typically takes several days for the pathologist to prepare and examine the tissue.

For superficial bladder cancers, a TURBT is a definitive procedure. Definitive means that it completely

Resectoscope

a specialized cystoscope-like device that is passed through the urethra through which one may remove bladder tumors by using a loop device that is connected to an electrical current.

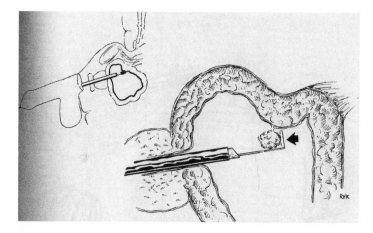

Figure 5   Resectoscope. This instrument is used to resect transurethrally or biopsy bladder cancer. Current *Genitourinary Cancer Surgery*, 2nd edition. Williams & Wilkins. Baltimore, MD, Ed. Crauford ED, Das Sakti 1997, page 347.

removes the tumor. For tumors that extend deep into the muscle of the bladder, TURBT allows for identification of the depth of invasion but is not definitive; thus, another type of treatment (surgery, chemotherapy, or radiation) will be required.

Most patients will not need to stay in the hospital overnight after a TURBT. The final decision on staying in the hospital or returning home is made based on the amount of resection necessary and the amount of blood in the urine after the procedure. These two factors will also determine whether a catheter needs to be left in place after the procedure, usually for a few days.

39. What are the risks of TURBT?

TURBT is generally regarded as a low-risk procedure. It is typically performed as a **day surgery** procedure, meaning that you will not need to stay in the hospital overnight. As with any surgery that requires anesthesia, a small risk is associated with the anesthesia. This risk is higher if you have other conditions such as asthma, **chronic obstructive pulmonary disease**, or **cardiovascular disease**, but is still generally very low risk.

The risks associated specifically with the TURBT procedure also are small. They include bleeding, infection, and bladder perforation. It is important to stop any "blood thinners" that are commonly prescribed for heart conditions, such as aspirin, Coumadin (warfarin), Plavix, and others. Ask your doctor about which of your medications you may need to stop taking before the procedure.

- Bleeding is the most common risk. The bladder is blessed with a rich blood supply, which facilitates

Day surgery

refers to a surgical procedure that is performed on the day of surgery but the patient goes home on the same day. It does not require an overnight hospitalization. It is also called an outpatient surgery.

Chronic obstructive pulmonary disease

a progressive disease that most commonly results from smoking, characterized by difficulty breathing, wheezing, and a chronic cough.

Cardiovascular disease

disease of the heart or blood vessels.

Treatment

quick and easy healing. During surgery, however, this creates opportunity for bleeding. After a TURBT, the urine is almost always light to dark pink. The color often will clear if you drink more fluid, thereby diluting the urine. Less commonly, blood clots will form in the bladder, which could block the flow of urine. In these cases, a catheter will need to be placed and the bladder irrigated with saline until the bleeding decreases. In a recent series of 2,821 patients who underwent TURBT, 2.8% (78 of the 2,821 patients) had problems with bleeding, and 3.4% (96 patients) required blood transfusion. **Straining to void** or move the bowels, deep coughing, or heavy lifting after the procedure may also increase the risk of bleeding.

Straining to void

the muscular effort used to either initiate, maintain, or improve the flow of urine.

- Urinary tract infections will occasionally occur after TURBT, although the risk is low. To minimize the risk, antibiotics are usually given at the time of the procedure. In patients who are at higher risk, a course of antibiotics may also be given after the procedure for a few days. Most infections that do occur can be treated with antibiotics at home, although rarely will an infection be serious enough to require intravenous antibiotics in the hospital. It is often difficult to diagnose an infection initially because surgery can cause the same irritative symptoms as an infection. If the symptoms get worse instead of better or fail to improve quickly, or if you develop a fever or cloudy urine, you should call your doctor.

- A bladder perforation occurs when the resection of the tumor extends through all of the layers of the bladder wall. In the study with 2,821 patients, 1.3% (36 patients) had small perforations in their bladders. A perforation usually occurs as a result of the urologist's need to resect deeply enough to remove the entire tumor. He or she must also include part of the wall of the bladder so that the pathologist can see how deep the tumor extends into it. Small perforations through the bladder wall heal quickly on their own. Until the perforation heals, a catheter will be left in place, usually for a few days. Larger perforations and those with continued leakage of fluid out of the bladder may require open surgery to close the hole. Complications are more likely to occur in patients who have larger tumors or multiple tumors.

- A TURBT is performed with the patient's legs raised in stirrups. This position is necessary to allow access to the bladder. Occasionally, this position can place pressure to a sensitive area that can cause blistering or numbness. These problems usually resolve on their own without need for other treatments.

40. What is perioperative chemotherapy?

Perioperative chemotherapy refers to the practice of instilling one of the bladder chemotherapies immediately after TURBT, usually while you are still in the operating room or the recovery room. Traditionally, these intravesical therapies have been given after the bladder has healed, 2 to 3 weeks after surgery. Several studies in the last 10 years have shown benefits to giving a single dose of chemotherapy at the time of TURBT. The benefit presumably derives from killing any cancer cells that are still swirling around in the bladder after TURBT, thus preventing them from implanting in the bladder.

Perioperative chemotherapy

chemotherapy administered shortly before planned surgery in hopes of improving local control and survival.

41. Who should get perioperative chemotherapy?

This question still creates some controversy. Based on the results of the studies, most experts recommend giving perioperative chemotherapy to almost everyone at the time of TURBT, unless the bladder is perforated during the surgery. The **efficacy** of all of the different agents seems about the same. We should point out that although most experts agree that perioperative chemotherapy is beneficial, its use has been slow to catch on among urologists in this country. A few experts feel that the benefit is small and therefore do not recommend its use. Thus, you should talk with your doctor specifically about this treatment if you are interested in it.

Efficacy

the power or ability to produce an effect.

42. What is photodynamic therapy?

Photodynamic therapy (PDT) is a new approach to bladder cancer treatment that uses a light source in the bladder to destroy cancer cells. One of several drugs is given to a patient intravenously. These drugs are designed to be absorbed more by cancer cells than by normal cells. The light source within the bladder is then activated. Exposure of the drug to light starts a chemical reaction that produces substances that are toxic to the cells, thereby killing them off. Because the tumor cells absorb more of the drug than normal cells, the tumor cells are preferentially killed.

Photodynamic therapy

cancer treatment that uses the interaction between laser light and a substance that makes cells more sensitive to light. When light is applied to cells that have been treated with this substance, a chemical reaction occurs and destroys cancer cells.

43. Who should receive PDT?

PDT is a new treatment that is still evolving. It is currently given only to patients with recurrent tumors who have failed BCG treatment. Newer sensitizing agents have improved its efficacy. In one study, 84% of patients with BCG-resistant papillary tumor had a complete response, and 75% of patients with carcinoma in situ had a complete response at the 3-month follow-up. At a median follow-up of 4 years, 31 of 34 patients who had responded were still tumor free.

Larger studies with long-term follow-up of patients are still needed before PDT becomes a mainstream treatment, but the early studies have shown great promise for this type of therapy.

44. What is the natural history of superficial bladder cancer?

Superficial bladder cancer is a recurrent and potentially progressive disease. Most studies have shown that patients with a higher stage and/or grade (Questions 29 and 30) have recurrences more frequently than do patients with a lower stage or grade. Approximately half of the lowest stage and grade tumors (Ta, Grade I/II) will recur, most of them in the first 3 months after treatment. Carcinoma in situ recurs in up to 70% of patients. Patients with multiple tumors or very large tumors are also more likely to have recurrences (up to 80%). Only 2% of patients with Ta, Grade I (the lowest stage/grade) will progress to a more invasive tumor, whereas almost half of T1, Grade III (the highest stage/grade superficial cancer) will progress.

45. How is carcinoma in situ treated?

The treatment of choice currently for carcinoma in situ is intravesical therapy with BCG (Question 35). Carcinoma in situ in most cases is not adequately treated by resection alone because it tends to be located diffusely throughout the bladder. Sixty to 70% of patients with carcinoma in situ will respond to a standard course of BCG. Although encouraging, this obviously means that 30% to 40% of patients will fail a standard course, and thus most experts advise further therapy. Some advocate two courses of BCG, whereas others prefer maintenance BCG for 3 years; urine is sent for cytology every 3 to 12 months. Also, periodic cystoscopy will need to be performed in the urologist's office, and any suspicious lesions will need to be biopsied and examined under the microscope by a pathologist.

Patients who fail to respond to BCG can be treated with other intravesical therapy. Interferon can be combined with BCG, or other chemotherapeutic agents like gemcitabine and valrubicin can be tried. If available, PDT can be considered (Question 42). Ultimately, patients in whom carcinoma in situ persists despite intravesical therapy should consider having a cystectomy.

46. How is urachal carcinoma treated?

The best course of treatment for urachal carcinoma is not clear because it is such an uncommon tumor. Patients with metastases are treated primarily with chemotherapy. Patients without metastases usually are treated with a partial cystectomy that includes removal of the tumor and bladder adjacent to the tumor along with the urachal ligament, including the umbilicus (navel). In addition to surgery, most patients are then treated with chemotherapy. There is no current consensus as to the best type of chemotherapy, but urachal carcinoma seems to respond better to treatments aimed at colon cancer than it does to treatments traditionally used in bladder cancers. Approximately half of patients will achieve 5-year survival if they do not have metastases. Many patients with urachal carcinoma will be eligible for **clinical trials** (Question 96).

47. Are there complementary or alternative therapies that are useful?

Most alternative therapies have not been well studied, making it difficult to recommend any specific therapy. Supplements like bovine and shark cartilage are often touted as being active against cancer, but no good studies have yet been completed that show a convincing effect. Herbal remedies are also available, although none have been proven to be effective. Any of these types of treatments can be expensive, and the dangers are equally unknown. To be effective against cancer, any treatment must be able to kill cancer cells. If an agent is potent enough to kill these cells, it should easily be able to kill normal cells and potentially have serious negative side effects. Be suspicious of treatments that allege results with no side effects. Furthermore, if you are on medications prescribed by your doctor, you need to be aware of the potential interactions between herbal therapies and those prescription medications.

In the end, we urge you to use caution and common sense when considering alternative therapies, especially dietary supplements and herbal medications. The National Institutes of Health maintains a web site of complementary and alternative medicine at *http://nccam.nih.gov/* that provides information and links to other resources. You can also see our appendix for more sources of information.

Clinical trials

a carefully planned experiment to evaluate a treatment or medication (often a new drug) for an unproven use.

Treatment

48. Do I need to seek treatment right away after being diagnosed with invasive bladder cancer?

Once you have been diagnosed with invasive bladder cancer, it is very important to seek treatment right away. The goal of bladder cancer treatment is to stop the cancer before it spreads outside of the bladder. Surgery can cure only when all of the cancer is removed. If the tumor has spread outside of the bladder, even in microscopically small amounts, then surgery will usually not be enough. A delay in treatment after your initial diagnosis may increase the risk that the tumor will spread outside of the bladder.

After diagnosis, several tests still must be performed before surgery. These tests are designed to help ensure that the cancer is confined to the bladder and that you are in optimal medical condition to get through the surgery. These tests must all be scheduled and performed and the results reviewed. This usually takes at least 2 or 3 weeks. Although the less time that elapses before surgery the better, it is generally agreed that the process should take less than 6 weeks to avoid significantly increasing the risk of spread. Thus, if you delay starting the process you will only add to the duration of time that passes before treatment. There is no need to panic, and remember that the process will usually take several weeks. However time is indeed of the essence.

PART FOUR

Intravesical Therapy

What is intravesical therapy?

What is the difference between therapeutic and prophylactic intravesical therapy?

What is immunotherapy?

More ...

49. What is intravesical therapy?

Intravesical therapy is treatment for bladder cancer that is applied directly to the bladder wall. It can be either **immunotherapy** or chemotherapy. The most common type of immunotherapy is BCG. BCG is immunotherapy that may be given with or without interferon. Several chemotherapeutic agents are also available, including mitomycin C, thiotepa, doxorubicin, epirubicin, valrubicin, and others. These are all administered directly into the bladder through a catheter. The medications are then able to act on the surface of the bladder without exposing the rest of your body to potentially harmful medications. (See Questions 51 and 64 for details on immunotherapy and chemotherapy.)

50. What is the difference between therapeutic and prophylactic intravesical therapy?

Intravesical therapy is said to be therapeutic when it is used to kill visible tumor cells. Some patients are unable to have their entire tumor(s) removed with TURBT because of the location or extent of the tumor. Intravesical therapy in these patients is designed to kill the remaining tumor and is thus called therapeutic. Intravesical therapy is also considered therapeutic when used to treat carcinoma in situ.

Many patients receiving intravesical therapy have already had their entire tumor removed by TURBT. The goal of this type of treatment is **prophylactic** (i.e., trying to prevent the growth of new tumors). Most experts believe that this type of treatment actually works not by protecting you from the development of

Immunotherapy

therapy designed to activate the body's own immune system to fight disease.

Prophylactic

preventive measure or medication.

new tumors, but by eradicating microscopic tumors that would eventually have grown into larger tumors.

51. What is immunotherapy?

Immunotherapy takes advantage of the methods used by our own **immune system** to attack cancer cells. There are two types of immunotherapy: passive or active. Passive immunotherapy involves the direct administration by doctors of molecules or cells to a patient and requires no involvement by the patient's own immune system. Active immunotherapy attempts to activate the patient's immune system to attack the cancer cells.

Immunotherapy could some day help to avoid the toxicity of chemotherapy and radiation for a variety of different types of cancers. For most cancers, this type of therapy is very new, and research is still ongoing. For bladder cancer, one type of immunotherapy, called BCG therapy, has been available for many years with excellent results.

52. What is BCG?

BCG stands for *Bacillus Calmette-Guerin*. It was developed in the 1920s. Some readers may recognize this as a vaccine for tuberculosis, as it is still used for this purpose in many countries. BCG is a live, **attenuated** (weakened) form of bacteria that causes tuberculosis. Although it is too weak to cause tuberculosis, it does activate the immune system. When it is given as a vaccine, it causes antibodies to be made that are active against the usual form of tuberculosis, thereby preventing most patients from acquiring the disease.

Immune system

the body system, made up of many organs and cells, that defends the body against infection, disease, and foreign substances. The immune system is often stimulated in specific ways to fight cancer cells.

Attenuated

to reduce in force, value, amount, or degree; to weaken. With respect to a bacteria/virus, to reduce the infectivity of a pathogenic microorganism.

Intravesical Therapy

Immune response

the body's response to things the body identifies as foreign or not normal.

For reasons that we still do not fully understand, the **immune response** to BCG is also able to kill bladder cancer cells. The bacteria attach to the urothelium and get taken up by the immune system. The immune system then actively destroys the cancerous cells in the bladder.

Immuno-compromised

a condition in which the immune system is not functioning properly.

Because it is a live bacteria, BCG should not be given to **immunocompromised** patients, that is, transplant recipients, HIV patients, patients taking prednisone, or patients with any other condition that may weaken the immune system. This is because immunocompromised patients would be at higher risk of developing tuberculosis. BCG should also not be given while there is gross hematuria because there is a higher likelihood of absorbing the bacteria.

53. Who should get BCG?

BCG is an option for treatment only after the initial TURBT has been performed and the pathologist has established a definitive diagnosis. Patients with low-grade, low-stage tumors are usually not given BCG. These patients have periodic cystoscopies performed to screen for tumor recurrence. If the tumor does recur in these patients, they are almost always low-grade, low-stage recurrences that are easily treated.

BCG is mainly aimed at those patients whom we believe are at more risk of tumor recurrence or progression. Patients with higher-grade, higher-stage tumors, patients with multiple low-grade tumors, patients with carcinoma in situ, and patients who have already had a recurrence should consider BCG treatment.

54. How effective is BCG?

BCG can best be described as *very* effective at preventing and delaying recurrences. Its actual effect depends on the grade and stage of tumor being treated as well as the dose and timing of the treatments. Most urologists will give weekly instillations of BCG for 6 weeks. Cystoscopy is then performed 6 weeks after the last treatment to look for tumor recurrences. Depending on the tumor pathology, your urologist may then elect to give you 3 more weeks of BCG at 3 months or a more aggressive regimen, repeating the BCG treatments every 6 months for 3 years. In patients who have a positive cytology after a full 6-week course of BCG, a second 6-week course of BCG may be necessary.

55. What are the risks of BCG?

BCG therapy is well tolerated by the majority of patients who receive it. It is, however, a live bacteria, and thus has a small potential of causing infection. Approximately 75% of the patients do complain of frequency and urgency immediately after the treatment, although this usually resolves quickly. Approximately 10% of people complain of some pain, which also quickly resolves. Twenty percent of patients will acquire a urinary tract infection unrelated to the BCG bacteria; this can usually be easily treated with a short course of antibiotics. Thirty percent of patients will have some bleeding after the treatment. About 25% of patients will experience mild flu-like symptoms of fever and achiness. The good news is that these side effects are usually short-lived and mild; thus, only 5% to 10% of patients will be bothered by the side effects enough to discontinue the treatment.

Symptoms such as a low-grade fever, chills, a flu-like malaise, and occasional joint aches are signs that the body is responding appropriately to BCG. If these symptoms are more than mild, they can also be a sign of serious infection by BCG. Fevers of more than 101.5, especially those that begin after 24 hours, persist more than 48 hours, or occur in the early evening, are more indicative of BCG infection. Patients suspected of having infection by BCG will usually be admitted to the hospital and treated with three antibiotics. Those who do not respond quickly may also be treated with steroids.

Prostatitis

inflammation of the prostate; may be infectious or inflammatory.

Approximately 1% will develop an inflammation of the prostate called **prostatitis**. This is usually treated with nonsteroidal anti-inflammatory medications such as ibuprofen, delaying treatments by 1 to 2 weeks, shortening the cycle of treatments, or antibiotics.

56. How is BCG given?

BCG is administered through a catheter. The nurse will ask you to urinate to empty your bladder completely. A urine dipstick test will be performed to test for blood or infection. If the dipstick test is negative, then the BCG will be instilled into your bladder though the catheter. Once the solution is in your bladder, the catheter will be removed, leaving the solution in your bladder. It is best to hold the medication in your bladder for about 2 hours. After 2 hours, you will urinate normally into a toilet (not outside or into an outhouse). Immediately flush the toilet and wash your hands.

The treatment course for BCG varies depending on the details of the individual tumor. A typical course is given once a week for 6 weeks, and then the cystoscopy exam is repeated. If the tumor has been eradicated, no further BCG is usually given at that time. Recurrent tumors are usually removed again by a TURBT. A second course of BCG may be given after this, with continued treatments possible in many cases.

57. What is interferon-α?

Interferons are chemicals that are part of your body's normal immune system. There are several subtypes of interferons, including α-interferon. BCG is, at least in part, effective against bladder cancer because it causes an increase of α-interferon in the bladder, which in turn helps to kill cancer cells. Interferon can be prepared and concentrated in a solution. Logically, by instilling it into the bladder, one could get a similar effect to BCG treatments with fewer side effects. Unfortunately, the effects of BCG appear more complex than just interferon.

When used alone, interferon initially performs about as well as BCG. Over time, however, patients treated with BCG have fewer recurrences, which indicates that the effect of BCG involves more than just activating interferon. The side effects of interferon are similar to those of BCG, meaning up to 27% of patients experience fever, chills, fatigue, and muscle aches (similar to having a mild flu).

Combining interferon with BCG is the most common way in which it is used today. Patients who have received BCG in the past but now have recurrences are often treated with combined interferon/BCG. Also, patients who have been unable to tolerate full-dose BCG can be treated with low-dose BCG combined with interferon with good effect.

Intravesical Therapy

58. What is mitomycin C?

Mitomycin C is a form of chemotherapy that is given intravesically in the same way that BCG is given. This type of chemotherapy acts by binding to tumor cell DNA, causing the DNA to malfunction or break apart. Without functional DNA, the tumor cells rapidly die.

59. How effective is mitomycin C?

The efficacy of mitomycin C, as with all intravesical therapies, depends on when and how it is given, as well as to whom it is given. Mitomycin C was initially given to patients who failed to respond adequately to BCG. Many of these patients did respond to mitomycin C, thus delaying or preventing the need for bladder removal surgery.

Many urologists now give mitomycin C immediately after TURBT in any patient who is at high risk for tumor recurrence. Its use in this setting has been found to reduce the frequency of tumor recurrence by 20% to 40%. It is especially effective in preventing early recurrence or those that occur in the first year. When a tumor is resected, cells are dislodged from the main body of the tumor. These cells swirl around in the bladder during the procedure and could potentially implant in other areas of the bladder, leading to recurrent tumors several months later. It is thought that giving a dose of mitomycin C as soon as the TURBT is complete can help kill the free cancer cells in the bladder, thereby preventing them from implanting and growing into recurrences.

60. What are the risks of mitomycin C?

When given intravesically, your body absorbs little or none of the drug, making systemic reactions rare. Allergic reactions can occur in 3% to 19% of patients.

Table 2   Common Intravesical Therapies for Bladder Cancer

Agent	Immunotherapy	Chemotherapy	Notes
BCG	Yes	No	Given once per week for 6 weeks
Interferon	Yes	No	Often given with BCG
Mitomycin C	No	Yes	Often given as single dose after TURBT
Thiotepa	No	Yes	

Rarely, some patients will experience decreased blood cell counts. Also, some researchers have reported a decreased bladder capacity (the volume of urine a bladder can hold).

The most common side effect is discomfort during urination (**dysuria**) and the frequent need to urinate (frequency). This can occur in as many as 41% of patients, but it usually goes away over a few days. Overall, most patients tolerate it very well and have minimal problems (Table 2).

Dysuria

pain or discomfort with urination.

61. What is bladder cancer surveillance?

Bladder cancer surveillance refers to the period of time after the bladder cancer has been removed or treated. It is a term that is used for patients who have been treated for superficial bladder cancer. Even after successful treatment of a tumor, it is important to remember that you are at risk of developing cancer in other areas of the bladder. The stage and grade of a tumor help to predict the risk of getting a recurrence, but in general, half of all patients will experience a recurrence. The term "surveillance" is usually applied only to patients who have superficial (not invasive) cancer

Intravesical Therapy

treated with a TURBT and/or BCG (or other intravesical therapy). We know that many patients will eventually have a recurrence of superficial tumors; thus, we must follow these patients closely. The need is similar to patients who have small skin cancers that have been removed; the cancerous growth has been removed, but the rest of the skin has had a lifetime of exposure to the sun and thus is at risk of developing a new cancer in a different area.

Although the exact timing of procedures for bladder cancer surveillance varies according to the type of tumor and physician preference, most patients will have a cystoscopy in the office every 3 months for the first year and will then decrease to twice a year or annually thereafter, as long as no new tumors are found. Also, urine cytology or other urine tests (see Questions 33 and 35) will be sent. Finally, remember that the ureters and kidneys possess the same types of cells as the bladder, and thus they too are at risk of a recurrence. Annual upper tract studies (Question 31) will also usually be performed for the first few years, with less frequent checks thereafter. Surveillance allows us to catch and treat any recurrence early on, with the goal of preventing progression to muscle invasion.

PART FIVE

Surgery

What is a radical cystectomy?

Who needs a radical cystectomy?

Should I have chemotherapy before
having a radical cystectomy?

More . . .

62. What is a radical cystectomy?

A radical cystectomy is the complete surgical removal of the bladder. It can be thought of as three separate procedures: (1) removal of the bladder, (2) removal of the lymph nodes, and (3) creation of a bladder substitute. When performed for bladder cancer in men, it usually includes removal of the prostate, **seminal vesicles**, and a portion of the **vas deferens**. When performed for bladder cancer in women, it usually includes removal of the uterus and cervix as well as the urethra, although the ovaries may be left in place. The urethra is removed in men only if the bladder cancer extends into it.

Another important part of the operation is called the pelvic **lymph node dissection**. This part of the procedure removes the lymph nodes through which the bladder drains. Remember that these lymph nodes are usually the first places where bladder cancer spreads. Taking the lymph nodes out allows us to do two things. First, looking at the lymph nodes under the microscope can tell us whether the cancer has spread outside of the bladder. Knowing this helps us predict the likelihood of the cancer coming back as well as help to direct any treatment in the future. Second, if the lymph nodes are the only place to which the cancer has spread, then removing the affected nodes may in fact cure you. For this reason, it is extremely important to have a thorough lymph node dissection performed.

Finally, remember that after the bladder is removed, your body still needs to store and drain the urine that it makes. The last part of the operation creates this new route for the urine. Several different options are

Seminal vesicles

paired glandular structures that are located above and behind the prostate gland. They produce fluid that is part of the ejaculate. They are removed during a radical cystectomy.

Vas deferens

a tubular structure that connects the epididymus to the urethra, through which sperm and semial fluid passes.

Lymph node dissection

in the case of bladder cancer, pelvic lymph node dissection, which is the surgical removal of the lymph nodes in the pelvis to determine whether the bladder cancer has spread to these nodes.

available, and you should discuss with your surgeon beforehand which one is right for you.

63. Who needs a radical cystectomy?

Radical cystectomy is the procedure of choice for many different types of patient. Most commonly, it is performed in patients who have muscle-invasive bladder cancer. If a bladder cancer invades the muscle, then other treatments such as TURBT and BCG are unlikely to fully treat the cancer, putting you at risk for metastases.

Although invasive cancer is the most common **indication** for a cystectomy, it is not the only reason. Carcinoma in situ has a high risk for progression to muscle-invasive cancer. Often, carcinoma in situ will respond to intravesical BCG or other types of intravesical treatments. Diffuse carcinoma in situ that persists despite treatment with BCG or other intravesical therapy should be treated with a radical cystectomy. This is because carcinoma in situ can become invasive and metastasize with few or no warning signs. It is also difficult or impossible to see during cystoscopy, making it difficult to monitor. These factors can lead to early cystectomy, done before the tumor becomes invasive in an attempt to prevent the cancer from spreading.

The last group of patients who may need a cystectomy is those patients whose tumors cannot be fully removed with a TURBT. There are occasionally patients whose anatomy makes it impossible to reach the entire tumor with the cystoscope. If the tumor cannot be eradicated with intravesical therapy, then they too may need a cystectomy despite only having superficial tumor.

Indication

the reason for undertaking a specific treatment.

Surgery

64. Should I have chemotherapy before having a radical cystectomy?

The answer to this question is still unknown. Some experts think that having chemotherapy before surgery can improve the long-term survival in some patients. It is difficult to say at this point that there is a definite advantage. Several studies have tried different combinations of drugs, but none has shown conclusively that patients receiving chemotherapy do better than those who just have surgery. A recent paper that combined all of these studies into one group did show a small increase in long-term survival. This small increase is only at the expense of exposing patients to the risks and side effects of chemotherapy. At this point, most patients do not receive chemotherapy before surgery, but it is an evolving area of research.

One important point to make about preoperative chemotherapy is that it delays surgery by several weeks while the patient receives treatment. There is a concern that some patients' cancer does not respond to chemotherapy. These patients might then have missed their window of opportunity to be cured by surgery because the chemotherapy treatments took several weeks to complete. It is not yet clear whether the benefits of the chemotherapy outweigh this potential risk.

65. Can I have surgery at my local hospital, or do I need to travel to a large referral center?

Many local hospitals across the country provide excellent care that is convenient for both you and your family. Several factors are involved in making this decision, but in the end, most patients make this type of decision based on (1) family support and (2) institutional and physician expertise. If the closest referral center is far away, it may be difficult or impossible for your family and friends to be there to support you around the time of surgery.

With that being said, it is your surgery and your future that are on the line; thus, you need to be certain that you can still receive high-quality care at your local hospital. This is rarely a clear decision from a medical standpoint and will usually boil down to your comfort with both your urologist and the local hospital.

If you would like to have surgery at your local hospital, it is important to be sure that the nursing staff is familiar and comfortable with the care that you will need after surgery or chemotherapy. The best and easiest way to assess this is to ask your doctor for the names and phone numbers of patients who have had the same treatments at that hospital and who would be willing to talk to you about their experiences.

Some patients may be concerned about going to a large referral center because they will be obligated to have residents (doctors in training) involved in their care. Although this is a valid concern, most patients find that these doctors in fact dramatically improve their care. Residents are at the hospital and are available to you 24 hours a day and are often able to spend more time with you than a local urologist who visits the hospital once a day. Again, talking to people who have had their treatment at that facility can provide valuable insight for you before making a decision.

66. What is laparoscopy?

Laparoscopy refers to surgery that is done by using instruments inserted into the body through a tiny incision. A camera attached to a small telescope inserted through another tiny incision provides visualization for the surgeon. This is one technique in a field that is now called minimally invasive surgery, or surgery that seeks to minimize the size of incisions as well as the manipulation of tissues necessary during conventional surgery. The major benefits in general are decreased blood loss, decreased postoperative pain, and an earlier return to work or normal activity.

Over the last 10 years, dramatic improvements in instruments and technique have allowed surgeons to perform virtually every type of surgery using a **laparoscope**. The first widespread use of the technique was to remove the gallbladder. Laparoscopic gallbladder removal can now be performed quickly and safely and is cost-effective for the healthcare system. This procedure is, however, relatively easy from a surgical standpoint. As more complicated procedures have been performed laparoscopically, questions have arisen as to their safety, speed, and cost. In surgery performed for cancer, questions arise as to whether the procedure can remove the cancer as effectively as traditional surgery. The answers to these questions for most procedures are that they are similar in safety, moderately to dramatically slower, and moderately more expensive. The cancer outcomes so far have been similar. Laparoscopy in bladder cancer remains an **experimental** procedure at this point, although it is being done successfully at some centers. Only a specialized, highly skilled laparoscopic urologist should perform the procedure at this time.

Laparoscopy

an operation that uses a laparoscope and other modified equipment that may be passed through very small incisions in the abdominal wall.

Laparoscope

a specialized tele-scope-like device that allows one to see into the abdominal cavity and pelvis through a very small incision.

Experimental

an untested or unproven treatment or approach to treatment.

67. Can a radical cystectomy be done via laparoscopy?

Absolutely. It *can* be done. Multiple surgeons have now reported that they have performed the procedure successfully. In women, the procedure technically is similar to removal of the uterus, a procedure that is commonly performed laparoscopically. In men, the procedure is complicated by the presence of the prostate attached to the bladder. Laparoscopic removal of the prostate, although uncommon, has now gained acceptance as a valid technique for removal of the prostate in patients with prostate cancer. Laparoscopic prostate removal takes significantly longer (4 to 8 hours) than traditional surgery (2 to 4 hours) and is more costly to the health-care system, but it does seem to provide some benefits to patients. These benefits mainly relate to a shorter hospital stay and shorter recovery period after surgery.

Laparoscopic removal of the bladder is a similar procedure, as the prostate is removed while still attached to the bladder. The creation of an ileal conduit or **neobladder** adds a significant new step to the procedure. Various techniques have recently been described to perform this portion of the procedure, but it remains a challenge undertaken by only a handful of surgeons in the world. In addition, the long-term outcomes in terms of cancer recurrence in these patients remain to be reported, although we expect it to be similar to traditional surgery.

Neobladder

an artificial/new bladder created by using a portion of the intestines that stores urine like a real bladder and allows one to urinate per urethra.

68. What is robotic surgery?

Robotic surgery is essentially an outgrowth of laparoscopy. Laparoscopy can be difficult because the instruments need to be long and straight to be

Surgery

inserted through the skin. It can thus be difficult to reach some areas and to manipulate the tissues appropriately (imagine trying to sew with chopsticks). Robotic surgery attempts to overcome these limitations. Miniaturized, motorized robotic arms are inserted into the body in the same way as the traditional laparoscopic instruments. The surgeon who is sitting across the room controls the arms. A camera is inserted in the same way as laparoscopy to provide visualization to the surgeon. The added flexibility of the instruments significantly decreases the difficulty of the procedures and therefore the amount of time it takes. Robotic surgery is still extremely expensive and is thus only available in a few centers across the country. Its use in bladder cancer surgery is therefore extremely limited.

69. I have had radiation treatments in the past. Can I still have a radical cystectomy?

Yes. The caution here is that radiation to the abdomen or pelvis (i.e., for ovarian cancer, prostate cancer, lymphoma, or other cancer) makes the procedure more difficult for the surgeon and increases the risks for the patient. Radiation causes the tissues to become very stuck together. In this situation, normal dissection during surgery is not possible, increasing the risk of inadvertently injuring normal structures such as the bowel or blood vessels. Also, prior radiation therapy decreases the body's ability to heal in those areas exposed to the radiation. This creates a greater risk of having leaks or other complications. Because of its increased difficulty and risk, a radical cystectomy after pelvic radiation should only be performed by surgeons with experience in this area. When performed by an experienced surgeon, the overall risk is about the same as for patients who have not had prior radiation, except that the risk of incontinence will be slightly elevated.

70. I am older person and am afraid that major surgery will be too much for me. Do older people do well after a cystectomy?

This is a valid concern and one that many physicians share. How old is too old? The answer here is encouraging. Two studies have looked at radical cystectomies performed in patients in their 80s. Both studies found that although there was a slightly higher risk of complications from the surgery, most of the increased risk was due to other illnesses. That is, a healthy 85 year old should do just as well as a healthy 65 year old. Older patients are more likely to have other medical conditions, such as heart disease or diabetes, that will add to the risk of the procedure. There is no such thing as too old. If you are relatively healthy and have a disease that could be cured by surgery, then you should discuss surgery in detail with your doctor.

71. What are the risks of a radical cystectomy?

A radical cystectomy is major surgery and as such has serious potential risks. Keep in mind, however, that the goal of surgery is to cure you of cancer. As such, minor complications are not uncommon, and major complications are possible. Up to one third of all patients will have at least one complication early on. You should talk to your doctor about the risks for you personally, as they vary greatly depending on your health and other medical problems. Not surprisingly, younger, healthier patients tend to have fewer problems than do older patients with more medical issues.

- Bleeding: As with any surgery, there is a risk of bleeding during the operation. Many patients will require blood transfusions. If for religious or personal reasons you cannot accept a blood transfusion, talk with your doctor directly before making a decision about the surgery. Some patients may be able to "donate" their own blood a few weeks before surgery. Then, if they require a blood transfusion, they can be transfused with their own blood.
- Cardiac: The surgery can often take 6 to 12 hours, during which time your heart must perform extra work. Most people will tolerate this easily, but a few (2% to 5%) will have heart problems such as congestive heart failure or even a heart attack. Your doctor and the anesthesiologist will evaluate you before surgery to minimize the risk and may even order heart tests such as echocardiograms, stress tests, or cardiac catheterizations to evaluate your cardiovascular status before surgery.
- Anesthesia: During the surgery, you will be under anesthesia with a tube inserted to breathe for you. Usually, this tube is removed at the end of surgery to allow you to breathe on your own. Sometimes this tube needs to stay in for a short period of time after the surgery, especially if you have a lot of extra fluid in your body or if you have a preexisting lung condition such as asthma, chronic obstructive pulmonary disease, or emphysema.
- Bowel: A piece of small or large intestine is used to make the bladder substitute. Your surgeon needs to repair the remaining intestine after this. It is a deli-

cate portion of the procedure, and this repair can occasionally (5% to 10%) leak or obstruct the intestine. These complications usually require a second operation, but some will heal without surgery. Also, anytime an operation is performed in the abdomen, scar tissue (adhesions) will form. These adhesions may sometimes cause pain or bowel obstruction months or years later.

- Urinary: Similarly, the new bladder substitute must be stitched together. Despite our best efforts, a few of these will leak urine. After surgery, you will have at least one or two drains left in place, and these drains are often enough to give the leak time to heal on its own. Rarely, if the leak fails to resolve, a second surgery can be required to fix it.

- Infection: Infections are not uncommon, although most can be treated with standard antibiotics. Infection can occur in the skin around the ostomy (**cellulitis**), deep in the abdomen or pelvis (**abscess**), or in the urine (urinary tract infection) or kidneys (**pyelonephritis**). Occasionally, a pocket of infected fluid will collect that needs to be drained by a small drain that is inserted through the skin in addition to using antibiotics. Urinary tract infections are common after a **urinary diversion** but tend to decrease over time.

- Deep venous thrombosis: After surgery, some patients will form blood clots in their leg veins, called **deep venous thrombosis**. The only symptom of this is swelling or soreness in the affected leg. If a piece of the clot breaks off, it will travel to the lungs and block the blood flow. This is called a **pulmonary embolus** and can be a life-threatening condition. While in the hospital, patients routinely

Cellulitis

an inflammation/infect of the skin and underlying tissue presenting with a warm, red swollen area.

Abscess

a localized collection of pus in part of the body.

Pyelonephritis

infection of the kidney, most commonly bacterial in origin.

Urinary diversion

a surgical procedure that diverts the flow of urine away from the bladder, typically to the abdominal wall, either directly by sewing the ureters to the skin or more commonly by sewing the ureters to a conduit; see *conduit*.

Deep venous thrombosis

blood clotting in the veins of the inner thigh or leg.

Pulmonary embolism

the obstruction of pulmonary arteries (arteries in the lungs) usually by detached fragments of a clot from a leg or pelvic vein.

have specialized devices placed on their legs that squeeze the calves, helping to prevent these clots from forming. An alternative to this is twice-daily shots of heparin. If a clot does form, you will need to be treated with blood thinners for several weeks.

Hernia

a weakening in the muscle that leads to a bulge.

Fascia

a fibrous membrane covering, supporting and separating muscles.

Incarcerated

with respect to bowel, bowel that is trapped, which may lead to swelling and decreased blood flow to the bowel segment.

Libido

sexual desire, interest in sex.

Dyspareunia

difficult or painful coitus (sex).

Erectile dysfunction

the inability to achieve and/or maintain an erection satisfactory for the completion of sexual performance.

- Hernia: A **hernia** is a weakening of the fibrous layer of the abdominal wall called the **fascia**. A weakness in the fascia can be seen as a bulging during straining. The abdominal contents that bulge into this pocket can occasionally become trapped or **incarcerated**. An incarcerated hernia is an emergency that needs to be treated with surgery. To avoid this situation, most hernias will need to be repaired with a procedure that places a synthetic mesh screen behind the fascia to reinforce it, preventing the bulging.

- Sexual dysfunction: This may affect both men and women after surgery. Women often experience decreased sexual desire (**libido**) or vaginal dryness because of hormonal changes and may have pain with intercourse (**dyspareunia**), especially early after surgery. In men, the incidence of **erectile dysfunction** after a cystectomy is similar to the rate after removal of the prostate for prostate cancer. In patients with normal erections preoperatively, up to 70% will regain erections after surgery if attempts are made to preserve the nerves going to the penis. Many men with bladder cancer already have some degree of erectile dysfunction, however, before surgery. The return of erections after surgery in these men will not be as good. The same options that are available to men with erectile dysfunction after prostate cancer surgery are available to men with erectile dysfunction after bladder cancer surgery (see Questions 75 and 76 for more details) (Table 3).

Table 3 Therapies for Erectile Dysfunction (for Questions 71 and 75)

Therapy	Dose	Timing of Use	Contraindications	Side Effects
Sildenafil (Viagra)	25–100 mg	0.5–1.5 hours before intercourse	Nitrite use, alpha-blockers within 4 hours, retinitis pigmentosa	Headache, dyspepsia, flushing, visual disturbance
Vardenafil (levitra)	10–20 mg	0.5–1.0 hours before intercourse	Nitrite use, alpha blockers retinitis pigmentosa	Headache, dyspepsia, flushing
Tadalafil (cialis)	10–20 mg	2 hours before intercourse. May last up to 36 hours	Nitrites, can use tamsulosin (Flomax)	Headache, dyspepsia, flushing, myalgias
Intraurethral Prostaglandin E1 (MUSE)	125–1,000 mcg	15 minutes before intercourse	Known hypersensitivity to prostaglandin E1 pregnant partner	Penile pain/burning, syncopal episode, priapism
Penile Injection Therapy (Caverject, Edex, Triple P)	Varies	15 minutes before intercourse	Those prone to priapism, Peyronie's disease	Pain, burning, hematoma, penile fibrosis
Vacuum Device	N/A	10–15 minutes before intercourse	Severe Peyronie's; use carefully with blood thinners	Penile pain, coolness, ejaculatory troubles, bruising
Prosthesis	N/A	Inflate just before	Requires surgery	Erosion malfunction infection

Any of these complications are made more common in patients with poor nutrition. To heal properly, the body needs a ready supply of energy and nutrients. In the days immediately after surgery, the bowels do not function, and you will not be allowed to eat. Most people will begin taking liquids again 3 to 5 days after the surgery. Your body has enough reserves for this amount of time. Some people, however, will take longer for their bowel function to return and may require intravenous nutrition (called **total parenteral nutrition**). In the weeks before surgery, it is very important to pay close attention to nutrition. Many patients benefit from protein shakes and other nutritional supplements.

Total parenteral nutrition

an intravenous form of nutrition that provides all essential nutrients.

Finally, there is the potential for complications further down the road. Most of these relate to the bladder substitute; thus, we discuss them in more detail when we go over each option.

72. What is a pelvic lymph node dissection?

A pelvic lymph node dissection is a procedure that removes those lymph nodes that are most likely to harbor metastatic bladder cancer. The lymphatic system collects fluid throughout the body and returns it to the bloodstream through its own set of tiny channels. Cancer cells often escape the bladder through these channels and establish sites of metastasis in the lymph nodes. If these lymph nodes are the only sites of metastasis, then we may be able to cure some patients of their bladder cancer. Removal of these lymph nodes also gives us important information to help direct any future treatments that may be necessary.

73. What are the risks of a pelvic lymph node dissection?

In most cases, pelvic lymph node dissection does not increase the **morbidity** of a radical cystectomy operation. This means that people who have a radical cystectomy with a pelvic lymph node dissection have the same outcomes from surgery as do those patients without the pelvic lymph node dissection. Rarely, a patient may develop a **lymphocele**. A lymphocele is a collection of the fluid that is normally drained through the lymphatic system. If this is very large or if it becomes infected, then it may need to be drained.

Very rarely, a nerve may be injured during the lymph node dissection. A nerve called the **obturator nerve** is most at risk during this procedure. The obturator nerve supplies some of the muscles of the thigh, often called the "tailor's muscles" because they are necessary when using the foot pedal of a sewing machine. Today, these muscles are used most often while driving an automobile to move the foot from the accelerator to the brake.

Finally, there is always a theoretical risk of injury to an artery or vein during the procedure. The pelvic lymph nodes are wrapped tightly around the arteries and veins and must be carefully removed. Although injury to these vessels does occur, it should be easily repaired during the surgery.

74. How long will it take to recover from a radical cystectomy?

Radical cystectomy with the creation of a urinary diversion is a major surgical procedure. It takes several hours to perform the procedure and includes operating

Morbidity

unhealthy outcomes and complications resulting from treatment.

Lymphocele

a collection of lymph fluid in an area of the body.

Obturator nerve

a nerve located on the pelvis that produces motor innervation to muscles in the thigh and skin sensation to the inner thigh.

Surgery

on the intestines. The recovery from this surgery can be expected to take much longer than shorter or less complicated procedures. Immediately after surgery on the intestines, their function is often not normal. It usually takes several days for bowel function to return. During this time, many surgeons place a **nasogastric tube** to drain the fluid that would otherwise accumulate and cause vomiting. The tube can usually be removed as soon as bowel function returns. The normal passing of gas best indicates the return of function. Once bowel function returns, a progressive diet will be tried. Clear liquids such as water, apple juice, Jell-o, or broth will be tried first. If these are well tolerated without nausea or vomiting, then about a day later solid food can begin again.

Nasogastric tube

a tube placed through the nose down the esophagus into the stomach to drain fluid accumulating in the stomach.

About a day or two after surgery, the nurses will help you to get out of bed, first to a chair but soon after to walk in the hallways. Pain control will be provided with intravenous medication until you are able to eat; then the intravenous medications will be stopped and **oral** pain pills will begin. You will be ready to go home when your pain is well controlled with only pills, you are able to walk on your own power at least from bed to the bathroom, and you can tolerate regular food. This usually takes 5 to 10 days if all goes well.

Oral

taken by mouth.

Some people, particularly those who are older or who have multiple other medical problems, may need to go to a rehabilitation facility after the hospital instead of returning directly home. This is to allow for physical therapy or nursing care that could not be provided at home. Once the patient's strength and healing has progressed sufficiently, he or she can then return home.

When at home, expect good days and bad days rather than a steady gain each day. You will initially tire very easily, and you may nap during the day more than usual. Your body is using a huge amount of your energy to repair itself after surgery, leaving little for your daily routine. For several weeks after surgery, you should not lift anything more than 5 to 10 pounds or do anything too stressful until the muscles and connective tissues have fully healed. It usually takes at least a month for your full energy to return.

Once you are completely healed, you will be able to resume virtually all of your prior activities. This usually takes about a month. Active patients who jogged, played tennis, golf, skied, or almost any other activity before surgery should be able to resume these activities in time. If you have a **urostomy bag** that you worry could become dislodged, then placing a loose binder around the abdomen can provide some relief of the concern. Before surgery, your doctor and/or an ostomy nurse will help choose a site on your abdomen for the **stoma** that will allow for easy access and optimal concealment. Those patients with a neobladder will initially find that they need to urinate frequently to prevent leakage. Over time, the neobladder stretches to accommodate larger amounts of urine, allowing longer times between voids.

Urostomy bag

a specialized collecting device that is applied to the urostomy stoma that collects urine.

Stoma

a surgically created opening in the skin for elimination of body waste, such as urine or stool.

75. How will having my bladder removed affect my sexual function as a man?

In addition to removal of the bladder, the procedure includes removal of the prostate and seminal vesicles. The portion of the procedure involving the prostate and seminal vesicles is essentially identical to that performed during a radical prostatectomy for prostate cancer. Thus, you share the same risks of erectile dysfunction after surgery as do men after prostate cancer surgery.

Over the last several years, techniques have been developed to preserve the nerves that travel next to the prostate on their way to the penis. If your surgeon is able to apply these techniques during your surgery, the odds of having a normal return of erections and orgasm is improved. The prostate and seminal vesicles produce the fluid that is ejaculated during orgasm, and thus there will never be a return of ejaculation. Additionally, because the vas deferens is cut during the surgery, no sperm will be ejaculated. Thus, even with normal return of erections and orgasm, it would be impossible to get your partner pregnant through intercourse. The testicles do continue to produce healthy sperm, however, making conception possible through in vitro fertilization. With modern techniques, sperm are removed from the testicle or **epididymis**, and eggs are removed from the woman. The egg is fertilized by the harvested sperm and reimplanted into the woman's uterus, allowing for a normal pregnancy thereafter.

Epididymis

a structure attached to the testes that stores sperm as they mature. Epididymis connects to the vas deferens.

Even without bladder or prostate surgery, erectile dysfunction is a very common problem. Fifty percent of men aged 40 to 70 are affected. Men with erectile dysfunction should talk to their doctor about the problem before surgery as well as after the recovery process. Fortunately, several easy options are now available to treat erectile dysfunction, including pills, intraurethral therapy, injection therapy, vacuum devices, and surgically inserted **prosthetics** (see Question 71) (Table 3).

Prosthetics

the art and science of making and adjusting artificial parts of the human body.

My husband had a radical cystectomy and an ileal conduit and had no evidence of any cancer outside of the bladder wall. We were so scared, and then so relieved to hear this information. As time went on and we resumed our normal daily routines and became comfortable with his stoma and the bag, we decided to resume sexual relations. Unfortunately, as a result of his surgery he couldn't get an erection. Our doctor had warned us about this, so we felt comfortable discussing it during one of our follow-up appointments. The doctor prescribed some pills, but these didn't work for my husband. He then tried injection therapy. This has worked. Although he would prefer not to have to give himself a penile injection, he finds that this option was better than the other ones that were described. We are now able to lead a complete life, similar to before the surgery.

76. How will a radical cystectomy affect my sexual function as a woman?

More attention has been focused on the effects of surgery on male sexual dysfunction than has been focused on female sexual dysfunction. Surprisingly, it is only in recent years that *any* attention has been focused here. In women, a radical cystectomy typically includes removal of the uterus (**hysterectomy**), ovaries and **fallopian tubes** (**salpingo-oophorectomy**), and a small portion of the vagina. The nerves that go to the clitoris and vagina are similar to those that go to the penis in men. Therefore, we can expect that a radical cystectomy may affect a woman's sexual function as well as a man's. If you are sexually active, it is important to discuss these issues with your urologist before surgery. **Nerve-sparing surgery** may be an option to help limit sexual dysfunction after surgery.

Surgery

Hysterectomy
removal of the uterus.

Fallopian tubes
two long muscular tubes that transport ova (eggs) from the ovaries to the uterus.

Nerve-sparing surgery
a surgical procedure for men with prostate or bladder cancer in which the prostate or bladder is removed and the nerves are left undisturbed with the goal of preserving erectile function.

In addition to producing eggs, ovaries also produce estrogen and testosterone. Testosterone is the dominant sex hormone in men, but is also produced in small amounts in women. It is known to be a driving force for a woman's libido (interest in sex). After removal of the ovaries, the levels of both of these hormones fall dramatically. Estrogen replacement after removal of the ovaries is common, although the risks and benefits are not entirely clear; thus, replacement therapy should be discussed with your urologist, primary care provider, or gynecologist. Testosterone replacement is also easily achieved with medications, but is still not well studied. If your libido is decreased after surgery, testosterone therapy may help it to return to how it was before surgery. Again, the risks and benefits of these therapies remain unclear, and thus each case needs to be addressed individually.

Some women may have difficulty with intercourse after surgery because of narrowing or shortening of the vagina. If you are sexually active before surgery and wish to remain active or even maintain the potential to be sexually active, it is important to discuss this with your doctor. During surgery, techniques to minimize the narrowing or shortening of the vagina can be employed to help preserve function and avoid potential pain with intercourse.

The nerves that supply the vagina, much like those that supply the penis in men, act to increase blood flow to the vagina when stimulated. The increased blood flow in turn stimulates vaginal lubrication. Therefore, any injury to these nerves during surgery can lead to vaginal dryness during sexual activity. For many women, this can be easily treated with the use of lubricants that are available at most pharmacies and supermarkets.

Researchers are now exploring the use of erectile dysfunction drugs in women. These drugs (Viagra, Cialis, and Levitra) are not currently approved for use in women and therefore are only being used in clinical trials.

77. Where will my urine go now that my bladder is gone?

This is an important question. Obviously, your body still needs to make urine. It would be ideal to replace your bladder with an artificial or synthetic bladder. Unfortunately, no one has found a man-made material that can be exposed to urine without becoming encrusted with stones. Any nonabsorbable synthetic material in contact with urine will cause stones to form. A single stitch in the bladder will quickly form a stone that in some cases can grow to the size of a football, completely filling the bladder. Until a synthetic material is found that will not form stones, we are forced to use other parts of the body that are available. The best substitute that we have found is a piece of your own intestine. Surgeons have successfully used portions of stomach, small intestine, and large intestine. In most cases, a segment of small intestine (the **ileum**) would be the best choice unless you had received prior pelvic radiation. In these cases, a piece of the large bowel would usually be best as it is less affected by the radiation treatments.

Ileum
a part of the small intestine.

As discussed in Question 2, placing tubes into the kidneys (nephrostomy tubes) or attaching to the ureters to the abdominal wall (cutaneous ureterostomies) are short-term options but not good long-term solutions. The ureters can also be attached to the colon

Surgery

Ureterosigmoid-ostomy

a specialized procedure whereby the ureters are connected to the sigmoid colon. Urine is thus evacuated with stools.

(**ureterosigmoidostomy**), allowing the urine to be passed during a bowel movement. This was a common procedure many years ago because it provided the ability for the patient to "hold and evacuate urine." Urine was voided with each bowel movement. Unfortunately, there is a high risk of colon cancer in patients who have had this type of diversion for many years. For this reason, it is now rarely if ever performed. The mixing of urine and feces in the bowel seems to be the cause of these cancers. Urine in contact with bowel separate from feces *does not* seem to have such an increased risk of colon cancer. Current techniques separate urine and feces so that your risk of cancer in the urinary diversion is significantly less than with a ureterosigmoidostomy.

Currently, most urologists will offer a patient who is having a cystectomy one of three options. The first and simplest option is called an ileal conduit (Figure 6). This uses a piece of the ileum to drain the urine to the skin, where it is collected in a bag. The ureters are attached to one end, and the other end is left open onto the abdominal wall. The urine then drains out of

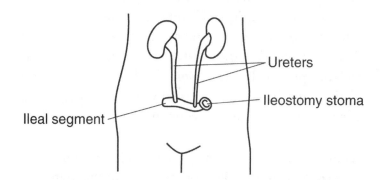

Figure 6   Ileal conduit urinary diversion. The ureters are sewn to a segment of bowel that is isolated from the remainder of the bowel. The end that remains in the body is closed, and the other end is opened to the skin, creating a stoma.

the open end and is collected by a urostomy bag. The patient needs only to drain the bag into the toilet every 4 to 6 hours. The bag can be worn under normal clothes, and thus no one needs know that you have a urostomy. Although it takes a little getting used to, almost all patients adjust to life with an ostomy bag quickly and easily and find that it does not interfere with their normal activities. Your urologist may be able to refer you to other patients who are living with a urostomy to get a firsthand account of how it will be.

The second option is to create what is called a continent urinary diversion. This is similar to the ileal conduit in that it is made out of a piece of bowel, but there is no ostomy bag. Instead, the urine is stored inside a pouch created from a segment of intestine. This is connected to the abdominal wall via a small channel, which is also created from the piece of bowel. The opening on the skin is then only about the size of a pencil eraser and does not protrude from the skin. Several times a day the patient needs to pass a small catheter through this channel into the pouch to drain the urine. It is a more complicated surgery to create the pouch and requires that you always carry a catheter with you, but it provides a way to avoid having a bag. If the pouch is not drained regularly, it can become overdistended and may even rupture.

The third and most complicated option is called a neobladder (Figure 7). It is an attempt to restore normal urination. Again, it is created with a segment of bowel, although it does require a much longer piece of bowel. As with the continent urinary diversion, your

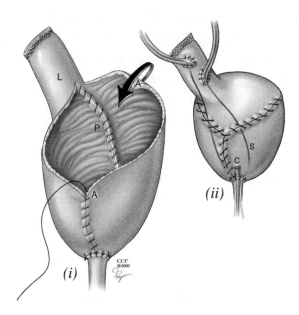

Figure 7   Orthotopic neobladder. The bladder is created from a segment of bowel that is reconfigured to create a pouch that is then sewn to the urethra to allow for storage and voiding. Used with permission from The Cleveland Clinic Foundation.

surgeon fashions into a reservoir that is able to store urine at low pressure. The ureters are connected to it in the same way as with the other two options. However, instead of connecting the pouch to the abdominal wall, it is connected directly to the urethra. This allows one to urinate as before the bladder was removed. Although this can be a great solution, it is not appropriate for every patient. The neobladder does not have the muscle that the normal bladder does, and thus it is unable to squeeze out the urine. One must learn to urinate by squeezing the other muscles in the abdomen to increase the pressure inside the neobladder (called **valsalva voiding**). The neobladder also lacks many of the normal bladder's mechanisms to

Valsalva voiding

use of abdominal muscles to increase bladder pressure to empty the bladder during voiding.

maintain **continence**, and some patients will be incontinent after the procedure.

78. How will I decide which urinary diversion option is best for me?

The most important part of the decision-making process is to talk with your urologist openly about your concerns. The two of you should decide together which option is best given any other medical problems, lifestyle, manual dexterity, and mobility, as well as the specifics of your tumor. A neobladder is often recommended for younger, healthier patients, although there is no age limit to the procedure. A neobladder requires a commitment by the patient to learning a new way to urinate, maintenance of a degree of physical fitness, and the ability to get to the bathroom at regular intervals. A neobladder is not appropriate in a patient who has poor mobility (i.e., after a stroke, spinal cord injury, severe arthritis, etc.). Patients who are not mobile or have other serious medical conditions or who just want the simplest option will do better with an ileal conduit. Obese patients and those who have had multiple abdominal surgeries or trauma may have a difficult time getting the ostomy bag to seal properly, causing leakage. A visit with a specially trained ostomy nurse can help decide the ideal location in these patients to ensure a proper fit of the bag.

A continent urinary diversion has become a less common choice since the popularization of the neobladder. A continent urinary diversion requires that a patient have adequate manual dexterity and strength to catheterize the pouch several times a day, every day for

Continence

with respect to urine, the ability to retain urine until a proper time to release it.

Surgery

the rest of their lives. Most patients who fit this category will be better served by a neobladder. Patients who have, for example, arthritis in their hands or poor vision may have a difficult time performing the catheterization, especially several years down the road. These types of patients again would be wise to choose an ileal conduit.

Although many physicians believe that an ileal conduit has the fewest complications, recent studies have not supported this. In fact, all three options have similar complication rates over the long term. Neobladders tend to have more problems early on, whereas ileal conduits develop problems later, which has likely led to the mistaken beliefs.

When I was diagnosed with bladder cancer, I was given the recommendation to have a radical cystectomy and an ileal conduit by my local urologist. I am a very active female who loves to travel. I still take care of myself by exercising and watching my weight. I used to smoke when I was younger but had quit many years before my diagnosis of invasive bladder cancer. The thought of having a stoma and wearing a bag was not a great option for me. I was middle age but didn't think that I acted old. I chose to get a second opinion to see if there were any other options for me and was offered the option of a continent urinary diversion, an Indiana Pouch. I catheterize the pouch several times a day to drain it. There is a very small opening on my abdomen through which I pass the catheter. I have no leakage of urine from the opening. The doctor who performed my Indiana Pouch had warned me that there were more complications associated with the Indiana Pouch, and I have experienced several. I developed a blockage where the ureter, the tube that drains my kidney, joins the pouch on each side; this required surgery. Despite these complications and the need for additional surgeries, I still am happy to not have to wear a bag.

79. What is a neobladder?

A neobladder is one of the options for reconstruction of the urinary tract after surgery. Other options include an ileal conduit or a continent cutaneous diversion. A neobladder is an attempt to replace the normal bladder as closely as possible with other tissues. A long segment of small bowel is isolated during surgery and fashioned into a bladder. It is then attached to the urethra to allow normal voiding after surgery. There is no bag on the abdomen and usually no catheterization is necessary.

I had a radical cystectomy and what my doctor calls a neobladder. They made a new bladder for me out a piece of my intestines. The new bladder is connected to my urethra so that I urinate through my penis. Urinating is different with the new bladder. I need to push the urine out using the muscles in my abdomen. I put myself on a schedule for urinating and find that if I drink alcohol I need to urinate more frequently to stay dry. If I decrease the amount of fluids I drink in the evening, I can stay dry at night by getting up only once at night. Before the bladder surgery I had to get up twice at night to urinate, so this is not much different.

80. What are the advantages and disadvantages of a neobladder?

The advantages of a neobladder over a urostomy or continent diversion are primarily lifestyle related and cosmetic. A neobladder is an attempt to replace the bladder with as close to a normal bladder, and therefore lifestyle, as possible. In an ideal situation, the neobladder will function like a normal bladder, storing urine at low pressure and forcing out urine on command by the patient. The most obvious advantage is that when all goes well there is no need for an external appliance or periodic catheterization. Patients with a urostomy need to wear loose-fitting clothing, but there are no such limitations with a neobladder.

The disadvantages to a neobladder are mostly *potential* disadvantages. That is, when the procedure goes well and everything works to its full potential, there is little or no disadvantage. Unfortunately, neobladders are prone to some problems that a urostomy is not. The most common potential problem is incontinence. About 90% of patients will be continent during the day, and 80% will be continent at night. This may mean that you will need to wear a diaper or pad if you have troublesome incontinence after surgery, especially at night.

In addition to incontinence, some patients will not be able to empty the neobladder completely when they void. This may mean that intermittent self-catheterization is necessary to empty the neobladder fully.

In order to make a neobladder that is large enough to hold urine for several hours, a longer segment of bowel is needed than for a simple ileal conduit. Patients who have certain bowel conditions may not be able to tolerate the removal of such a large piece and would do better with a short ileal conduit.

Intestine normally secretes a large amount of mucous. When separated and used as a neobladder, the mucous production generally decreases over time. Some patients will continue to produce mucous, which can accumulate and obstruct the flow of urine or cause stones to form. These patients will need to place a catheter into the neobladder and irrigate it free of mucous periodically.

A continent, catheterizable diversion often has a relatively high rate of complications in the first 1 to 2 years. Most of these are related to narrowing of the channel through which the catheter passes, however, and are relatively easy to treat with minor procedures. Only about 2% will fail completely and need to be converted to a urostomy with a bag, whereas about 5% will have problems with leakage of urine. About 10% will experience complications several years later, including stones, hernias, and bowel obstructions. As with a neobladder, a larger segment of intestine is required to create this type of diversion. Some patients may continue to have troublesome mucous production inside the diversion, requiring daily irrigation to prevent mucous plugs, stones, and infections.

Most studies that directly compare the **quality of life** after surgery have found that patients are mostly very satisfied with either choice. These studies have shown that neobladder patients are no more or less satisfied than patients with a urostomy bag. Also, the overall complication rates between the two are similar, although each has its own associated types of complications. Thus, it is important to review carefully the advantages and disadvantages of each to decide which will suit your lifestyle the best.

Quality of life

an evaluation of healthy status relative to the patient's age, expectations, and physical and mental capabilities.

81. How will I manage a urostomy?

Removal of the entire bladder, radical cystectomy, is the gold standard treatment for invasive bladder cancer. Rarely, individuals may be candidates for less invasive surgery or bladder-sparing regimens. Historically, the primary option to divert the urine after a radical cystectomy was an ileal conduit (see Question 77). Over the years, a variety of continent urinary diversions and "neobladders" (see Questions 77 and 79) have been developed in an effort to allow people to feel as "normal" as possible. In some individuals—that is, those who lack manual dexterity, who are dependent on caregivers—an ileal conduit is the most appropriate form of urinary diversion. In others, the surgeon may recommend an ileal conduit, or the patient may choose an ileal conduit.

Colostomy

the surgical construction of an "atypical anus" between the colon and the surface of the abdomen.

As with a **colostomy**, an ileal conduit has a nipple-like opening on the anterior abdominal wall (the belly) through which the urine passes into a specially designed collecting bag. Periodically throughout the day the bag is emptied. In the evening, extension tubing may be connected to the bag to allow the urine to drain continuously into a larger bag to prevent the bag from filling to capacity at night.

Several worries and concerns come to a patient's mind when an ileal conduit is proposed or discussed: (1) How will the ileal conduit change my body appearance, or will my spouse find me unattractive? (2) Will others be able to detect that I have a bag; that is, will it show through my clothes, and will it smell? (3) Do the bags leak?

The surgery to remove your bladder requires an abdominal incision. Typically, this will heal as a pencil thin line that runs up and down the middle of your abdomen. In select institutions, surgeons are performing the surgery via a laparoscopic approach to allow for a smaller surgical incision and ideally a quicker recovery. Thus, you will already have a small change in your physical appearance related to removing the bladder. The size of the stoma and the location of the stoma will vary with the segment of bowel used to make the urostomy. Typically, a segment of small intestine, ileum, is used. The ileum, smaller than the colon and often the size of the stoma, is smaller than a half-dollar coin. The ileum is mobile, and this allows the surgeon to locate the stoma where it will be easiest for you to access and be most comfortable. Often, you will meet with a stoma therapist before your surgery, and this individual will select the most appropriate site(s) for your stoma location depending on your body habitus, where the waist of your pants/skirts falls and the segment of bowel that the surgeon plans to use. Ileal conduit stomas tend to be located lower in your abdomen than those derived from a segment of the large intestine. The large intestine is often used for a urostomy in individuals who have a history of prior pelvic radiation because it is the segment of bowel that is least likely to have been damaged by the radiation treatments.

There are two components of the drainage system: (1) an adhesive wafer with a circle the size of the stoma cut out of it that adheres to the skin around the stoma and (2) the collection bag that snaps onto the wafer with a water-tight seal. The wafer also protects the surrounding skin from irritation from the urine. The bag is flat, so it is not discernible in your clothing unless it is very full and your clothing is tight. The collection system is designed to be watertight. Leakage may occur if you fail to secure the bag to the wafer correctly or if you do not close the drainage port at the bottom of the bag properly. Because it is common to make more urine at night, an extension tube may be connected to the bottom of the urostomy bag and to a larger collection bag to avoid having to awaken at night to empty the bag.

I had a radical cystectomy and an ileal conduit. The stoma therapist saw me before my surgery and marked the best location for the stoma. After the surgery I wanted to resume my golf and tennis activities, but I was so afraid the bag would pop off and I would be soaked in urine. My wife sews a lot and came up with a great idea. She made a pocket in my boxer shorts. I could put the stoma bag into the pocket, which prevented it from flopping around. It has worked out great. Now I am playing golf, tennis, even swimming.

82. How will a bag on my abdomen affect my lifestyle?

Having a bag on your abdomen will not prevent you from doing the things that you used to do before surgery. The bag is pretty secure when snapped onto the wafer properly. Some individuals who are very active may use a strap or something of that nature to lightly press the bag against the skin to prevent it from moving about during strenuous activity. As one patient just described, his wife sewed a pocket into his underwear to hold the bag so that it would not move around while he golfed and played tennis. You can even swim with the urostomy bag. The adhesive used to secure the wafer is quite strong.

With the stoma therapist, it is important that you identify the waistband of your sports clothing so that he or she can place the stoma in a location where both it and the bag will be covered.

83. What are the possible long-term problems with a urostomy?

Long-term problems after an ileal conduit are not uncommon. Overall, up to two thirds of patients will experience some type of problem. These problems can be categorized as follows.

Stoma: About one in four patients will have a problem related to their stoma. The most frequent problems are parastomal hernias (a weakening of the tissues around the stoma, allowing the intestines to bulge around it), **stomal stenoses** (narrowing of the opening of the stoma), and irritation/bleeding. If the appliance does not fit properly, the skin surrounding the stoma may become irritated and prone to yeast infections. The majority of these occur during the first few years after surgery.

Bowel: A similar number of patients (about 25%) will have problems related to their bowels. These problems include bowel obstruction, diarrhea, and **fistulae**.

Infection: Urinary tract infections and/or kidney infections occur in 5% to 10% of patients in the first few years after surgery. Most of these infections are not serious and can be easily treated with antibiotics, but a few patients will get serious or recurrent infections.

Stomal stenoses
narrowing of the stoma.

Fistulae
abnormal passages or communication between two internal organs or leading from an internal organ to the surface of the body.

Urinary obstruction: About 10% of patients will have a **stricture** of the connection between the ureter and the conduit. These strictures can block the drainage of urine from the kidneys, causing obstruction. They often require a second surgery or placement of stents to unblock the kidneys.

Stricture

scarring as a result of a procedure or an injury that causes narrowing.

Stones: Some patients will develop kidney stones several years after the procedure. The rate rises over time, and up to 40% of patients may have a stone at 10 years after the procedure.

Electrolyte disturbances: The bowel has evolved to absorb nutrients and to secrete waste products from the system. Although this is advantageous in the usual setting, it can be problematic when we reassign it to carry urine. When the bowel is exposed to urine, it may over-absorb salts and acids that the kidneys have secreted. This can usually be corrected with medications. Continent diversions and neobladders have urine exposed to the bowel for longer periods of time and thus are more prone to these types of problems than are ileal conduits.

84. What is a continent urinary diversion?

A continent urinary diversion provides a reservoir for the urine that can be drained every few hours by a catheter inserted by the patient. A segment of bowel is used to create a pouch inside the abdomen into which the urine drains. A small channel is then created that connects the pouch to the abdominal wall. This channel has a valve mechanism that prevents the urine from leaking. The channel is just large enough for a small catheter to be passed through it into the pouch. The pouch must be drained every 4 hours or so to prevent it from becoming overdistended. Overdistension can cause leakage or even rupture of the pouch.

Because the pouch is made of intestine, it may develop a buildup of mucous. To prevent this, it may need to be irrigated regularly with saline. Continent urinary diversions are associated with stone formation. Because the entrance to the pouch is through only a long, narrow channel, treatment of the stones can be difficult. Other risks include obstruction where the ureters are attached to the pouch and stricture or damage to the catheter channel, requiring surgical revision.

The advantages of a continent urinary diversion include not having a bag on the abdomen and a small stoma that is flush with the skin. Thus, it is cosmetically more appealing to some patients.

85. What is a partial cystectomy?

A partial cystectomy is the removal of only that part of the bladder that has cancer in it. It essentially takes the place of the TURBT in other bladder-sparing **protocols**. It potentially improves the removal of the tumor over TURBT and gives the pathologist a better ability to identify the tumor and its limits correctly because the entire tumor is removed in one piece. It is often, although not always, combined with chemotherapy.

Protocol

research study used to evaluate a specific medication or treatment.

86. Who is a candidate for a partial cystectomy?

To be eligible for a partial cystectomy, the tumor must be just in the right place and just the right size. Tumors at the dome (top) of the bladder are the most amenable to partial cystectomy. Many patients without cancer develop outpouchings in their bladder called a **diverticulum**. These outpouchings have no muscle on them, but they still have the ability to develop tumors like the rest of the bladder. Patients with a tumor in a diverticulum are particularly good candidates for partial cystectomy because of the difficulty of removing the tumor with a TURBT. Overall, however, only 5% to 10% of patients will have tumors that are appropriate for partial cystectomy. The presence of carcinoma in situ or multiple small tumors usually would make one ineligible for this procedure. This refers to those patients with transitional cell cancer, which is the vast majority of patients. Partial cystectomies are more often performed for other types of bladder cancer, especially in children with cancers involving the bladder.

Diverticulum

in the bladder, a small sac-like structure that lacks a muscular coat and thus does not contract like other areas of the bladder.

87. What are the risks of a partial cystectomy?

The immediate surgical risks of a partial cystectomy are similar to the risks for a radical cystectomy. These include bleeding, infection, damage to adjacent organs, and so forth (see Question 39). During a radical cystectomy, the bladder is removed intact. For a partial cystectomy, the bladder is opened, which potentially exposes the body to a risk of spread of the tumor during surgery. Current precautions taken during partial cystectomy seem to avoid spreading the tumor, but there is some theoretical risk. Another added risk to a partial cystectomy is the potential to have a recurrence of the bladder cancer in a new area of the remaining bladder. This is a life-long risk for those who have had a partial cystectomy, requiring frequent cystoscopy and cytology to monitor for any recurrence. At least 40% of patients will eventually have a recurrence.

88. What is a ureteral stent, and how is it put in?

A **ureteral stent** is a long, soft tube that stretches from the kidney to the bladder. You have probably heard about cardiac stents for people who have clogged arteries. These stents hold the arteries open so blood can continue to flow to the heart. Ureteral stents are similar in that they allow the urine to drain through the ureter if there is some type of blockage. Urologists place stents for many common types of blockages, that is, from a kidney stone, scarring, or occasionally a tumor. If the blockage is severe, it can cause the urine to back up into the kidneys. There are oftentimes no symptoms when this happens because it occurs very slowly over time. If it happens quickly, there may be some back pain on the side that is blocked. Complete blockage will cause the effected kidney to stop working until the obstruction is relieved. Long-term obstruction can permanently damage a kidney. Finally, if both kidneys are blocked, then the patient will develop renal failure.

Ureteral stent
a plastic tube that is used to keep the ureter open and allow for the drainage of urine.

When ureteral obstruction is present, the first approach is usually to place a stent to bypass the obstruction. The stent is put in with the patient under anesthesia in the operating room. A cystoscope is used to place the stent. A wire is passed through the ureteral orifice and advanced into the kidney. The stent then slides over this wire and is pushed all the way into the kidney. An X-ray machine in the operating room shows us how far up to slide the stent. The wire is then removed, leaving one end of the stent in the kidney and the other end in the bladder. The urine now has a clear path all the way down, and the kidney should quickly recover its function.

Occasionally, it is impossible to get a wire into the ureter from the bladder because of a severe obstruction or obliteration of the opening by a tumor. In these cases, the procedure will be aborted without a stent being placed, requiring an alternate type of drainage. To relieve the obstruction, an interventional radiologist will place a nephrostomy tube into the kidney through the back. The radiologist will usually again try to place a stent, this time by passing a wire from the kidney down to the bladder with the guidance of an X-ray. If the radiologist is able to get the wire past the obstruction, then he or she will pass a stent over the wire and leave the nephrostomy tube in place. A few days later the tube can then be removed if the stent is functioning properly. Rarely, a stent will be unable to relieve the blockage, and an alternative such as a nephrostomy tube or surgery will need to be considered.

Although stents work very well to relieve obstruction, they do have a downside. To hold the stent in place, it has a curl at each end. When the bladder is full, the curl floats away from the wall of the bladder. When the bladder is empty, however, the curl will often bump against the wall of the bladder causing irritation and spasm. Some people will also experience an ache in the kidneys from the curl hitting the wall there. The discomfort of the stent will often improve within the first week. There are also antispasm medications that may help improve the symptoms.

Over time, any foreign material in contact with urine will tend to develop stones. To prevent this, stents need to be removed or changed within 4 to 12 months. If you have a stent, be sure to remind your urologist to schedule you for these changes.

Surgery

PART SIX

Nonoperative Therapy

What is bladder-sparing therapy?

What are the risks of bladder-sparing therapy?

What is gene therapy, and is it available
for bladder cancer patients?

More ...

89. What is bladder-sparing therapy?

Bladder-sparing therapy refers to any approach to the management of muscle-invasive bladder cancer in which the goal is to avoid radical cystectomy. There are a variety of approaches, mostly based on the use of chemotherapy and/or radiation combined with transurethral resection of the tumor. In the past, chemotherapy or radiation therapy used without surgery was tried, but the results were poor. Combining chemotherapy, radiation therapy, and surgery allows some patients to avoid complete removal of their bladder. Although there has been success using this type of treatment, standard care for muscle-invasive bladder cancer remains removal of the entire bladder (radical cystectomy), with chemotherapy reserved for patients whose cancer could not be completely removed. Of those patients embarking on bladder-sparing therapy, only 40% ultimately have their bladder saved.

*I was scheduled to have my bladder removed and was admitted for my preoperative preparation. As I started to drink the fluid that they gave me to help clean out my intestines, I became more and more anxious about the upcoming surgery. That evening I decided that I could not go through with the surgery. I was too worried that something terrible would happen to me and that my poor wife would be left alone to take care of our children. I just couldn't do it. I told the nurses, and they called my urologist who came in to talk to me. She told me that a radical cystectomy was the best option for me, but when she realized that there was no way I was going to proceed with it, she discussed the option of chemotherapy and radiation therapy. Since it was late at night, she had me stay overnight, and the next morning I talked with the oncologist and the **radiation oncologist**. The chemotherapy and radiation therapy worked for me. The urologist re-biopsied the area where my*

Radiation oncologist

a physician who treats cancer through the use of radiation therapy.

tumor was and could find no evidence of any residual can-
cer. I have had several CT scans that have been normal,
and I have periodic cystoscopies. I am several years out and
realize that I took a risk not having my bladder removed,
but so far I have done well.

90. What are the risks of bladder-sparing therapy?

Bladder-sparing protocols have largely shown similar
rates of long-term survival compared with immediate
cystectomy. The studies have been criticized, however,
as falsely improving their results by selecting only
those patients who were already likely to do well. This
could mean that there is in fact a survival advantage to
having immediate surgery rather than waiting until
after a trial of chemotherapy. Patients who show evidence of tumor recurrence on these treatments will
usually then undergo a radical cystectomy with urinary diversion. There have been concerns raised by
some experts that the delay in time to radical cystectomy while having chemotherapy may increase the
risk of metastases significantly, but definitive data on
this do not exist.

Another disadvantage to these treatments is that they
are very complex and require close cooperation
between several specialists and a commitment on the
part of the patient. This means that they can be offered
only at a few specialized centers and only to a few
patients. Even in those patients who successfully **salvage** their bladder with these treatments, some will
have decreased bladder capacity or suffer from severe
urgency after treatments. With the advent of new techniques to create a neobladder, most patients who could

Salvage

a procedure intended
to "rescue" a patient
after a failed prior
therapy.

complete the bladder-sparing protocol would do as well or better with immediate surgery and neobladder.

91. What is gene therapy, and is it available for bladder cancer patients?

If we know that bladder cancer results from damage to a cell's genes, can't we just fix the genes? There has been much excitement in recent years about our growing understanding of genetics and the potential to use "gene therapy" to cure a variety of diseases, including cancer. Although gene therapy is not currently advanced enough to treat bladder cancer, many people are working very hard to make it a reality.

The ability to treat bladder cancer with gene therapy is hindered by two basic problems. First, in order to "cure" the cancer, the genes must be inserted into every cancer cell. This is an unrealistic goal, but a less than 100% effect could still be helpful to patients. Second, there is not just a single genetic problem that causes bladder cancer. Bladder cancer results from damage to multiple genes, but not necessarily the same genes in each patient. This makes gene therapy exponentially more difficult.

Several strategies are now being pursued to make gene therapy a reality. The most promising are to use gene therapy in addition to current treatments. The goal will not be to cure the cancer directly but rather to amplify the normal response to treatment such as BCG, radiation, or chemotherapy. Early trials have shown that the approach is feasible, although several technical barriers must be overcome before it is approved for general use.

PART SEVEN

Metastatic Disease

How does bladder cancer spread
outside of the bladder?

If bladder cancer does spread, where
in my body will it go?

Are there any blood tests to check for
the spread of bladder cancer?

More . . .

92. How does bladder cancer spread outside of the bladder?

Whether bladder cancer is superficial or invasive, it must still be confined to the bladder to be treated successfully by surgery. Once the tumor escapes from the bladder, it is difficult or impossible to remove the tumor completely. Like any other cancer, bladder cancer has three different routes by which it can escape the confines of the bladder. These three are (1) direct extension, (2) lymphatic spread, and (3) vascular spread.

1. Direct extension: As the tumor grows, it may gradually extend through each layer of the bladder wall. Once it has grown through the entire bladder wall, it may continue to grow directly into an adjacent structure, such as the rectum, prostate, vagina, or uterus. When your doctor performs a rectal exam, he or she is checking for this type of growth. By pushing on your abdomen at the same time, he or she can determine the extent of the spread. Women with bladder cancer should also have a pelvic exam as part of the evaluation to check for growth into the vagina or uterus. If the tumor has invaded into adjacent organs, then surgery will not often be curative, and your doctor may recommend alternative treatments. The amount of extension is assessed by a combination of the tumor biopsy, physical exam, and a CT scan.

2. Lymphatic spread: This is usually the first way in which bladder cancer spreads. In addition to blood vessels, the body has a second network of channels to collect fluid. This is called the lymphatic system. The main job of this system is to carry fluid and cells back to the bloodstream.

The lymphatic channels carry the fluid to the lymph nodes. These lymph nodes play an important role in your immune system, but they also give tumor cells fertile islands on which to grow. The natural environment of these islands provides everything a tumor cell needs to prosper. Once a node has been seeded with tumor cells, it will enlarge and can eventually obstruct the flow of lymph. Most importantly, it signals us that the tumor has spread outside of the bladder, which will influence the types of treatment your doctor can offer you. Many urologists feel that removal of all the lymph nodes with cancer in them can improve long-term survival in these patients. If you are having surgery, discuss with your doctor how extensive the lymph node part of the surgery will be.

3. Vascular (bloodstream) spread: If the tumor grows into a blood vessel, then cells can be swept into the bloodstream. They will circulate in the blood until they die, are removed by your immune system, or land in another organ and begin to grow. The most common locations for blood-borne bladder cancer cells to land are the liver (38%), lung (36%), bone (27%), adrenal glands (21%), and intestine (13%). Less commonly, it may spread to the other organs. Squamous cell cancers are the most likely to go to the bones.

93. If bladder cancer does spread, where in my body will it go?

The spread of any cancer outside of its organ of origin is called a metastasis. Bladder cancer tends to metastasize first to the lymph nodes in the pelvis. This is why the lymph nodes are removed during surgery. Some surgeons feel that removal of these lymph nodes only provides information to doctors and patients about the extent of disease. Recently, however, other surgeons have reported that some patients can be completely cured of their cancer by removing all of the affected lymph nodes. This idea remains under investigation, but many surgeons are now performing more extensive lymph node removals with the hope of improving survival.

Other sites of metastases for bladder cancer include lung, brain, liver, and bone. Lung metastases often cause shortness of breath, chronic cough, or blood in the sputum. Brain metastases often cause prolonged headaches. Liver metastases can cause more vague symptoms such as weight loss, appetite loss, fever, or easy fatigue. Bone metastases can often be painful but can also weaken the bones and can cause the bone to fracture easily.

Bladder cancer metastases can be treated with various combinations of chemotherapy with or without radiation. A few patients will also require surgery to improve the symptoms associated with some sites of metastases, that is, to stabilize a weakened bone.

94. Are there any blood tests to check for the spread of bladder cancer?

Some cancers produce specific substances that can be measured in the blood. Many readers will be familiar with the relationship of PSA to prostate cancer. After surgery for prostate cancer, the blood levels of PSA should decrease to zero. By periodically rechecking the level of PSA in the blood, we can monitor for a recurrence of the prostate cancer. Tumors from some other organs have different markers that can be followed by blood tests. Bladder cancer, unfortunately, does not have a useful marker like PSA. There is of course great interest in discovering and developing a blood test that could give us this information, but it has not yet been identified. We rely instead on other clinical information to check for the spread of cancer, especially X-rays and CT scans.

95. How is metastatic bladder cancer treated?

Metastatic bladder cancer is generally quite difficult to treat. Current treatment for bladder cancer that has spread outside of the bladder is aggressive chemotherapy. Most often, a combination of four drugs is given. These medications are abbreviated M-VAC, which stands for *m*ethotrexate, *v*inblastine, *a*driamycin (also called doxorubicin), and *c*isplatin; 60% to 70% of tumors will respond to this regimen, although complete responses are only seen in about 30%. Of the 30% who achieve a complete response, almost all will eventually relapse. This type of chemotherapy may be difficult for some patients to tolerate, and the number of patients who do not respond is significant. Researchers have therefore had great interest in devising a more effective, better tolerated regimen since M-VAC was first used 15 years ago, but no therapy has proven better.

One trial has, however, shown similar results using a less toxic regimen of two, called gemcitabine and cisplatin. Some oncologists are now recommending this newer regimen because it is better tolerated with similar results. New drugs and new combinations of existing drugs are constantly being evaluated in clinical trials that may be appropriate for some patients.

Recently, some patients with metastatic bladder cancer have been treated with a combination of chemotherapy and surgery. The metastatic tumor was completely removed by surgery, with chemotherapy given in addition. Early results of this approach are promising, but the treatment is only being done as part of a clinical trial until a definite improvement can be shown.

96. What are clinical trials?

A clinical trial is the process through which new medications or therapies are tested to determine their ability to perform their stated task. They are also used to evaluate surgeries, radiation, and combinations of these treatments. Not all trials lead to success, but many do. There are four phases of clinical trials.

Phase I: This is the first way in which a new treatment is tested with humans. Before a phase I trial, the treatment is researched in the laboratory until it is believed to be safe and effective. Phase I trials test the treatment on a small group of patients who have failed standard therapies. The goals of phase I are to determine the anticancer activity of the treatment, the effective dose, and identify any unexpected side effects. The dose is initially very low and then slowly increased if it appears safe.

Phase II: If a treatment passes phase I, it can be tested in a phase II trial. These trials are usually still limited to those patients who have failed conventional therapy.

The goal of these trials is to identify the effectiveness of dosages, and they use a larger number of patients.

Phase III: In these trials, the new treatment is tested against standard therapy. Volunteers are **randomized** to receive either the new treatment or standard treatment, and neither the patients nor the doctors should know which treatment is given until after the study and whether it is feasible. Two separate, successful phase III trials must be completed before the treatment is eligible for **Food and Drug Administration** approval.

Phase IV: After a medication is approved by the Food and Drug Administration and made available to all patients, it continues to be monitored in a phase IV trial. Uncommon side effects may be identified as the number of patients increases and the types of diseases treated change.

97. How do I get involved in a clinical trial?

Most patients become involved in a clinical trial at the invitation of their own physician. Even at the largest centers, any individual physician will be involved in only a small number of trials, which may or may not apply to you. With the advent of the Internet, it has become dramatically easier for patients to find clinical trials themselves. This is potentially a tremendous opportunity, but with it comes potential dangers for a partially informed patient. Before deciding to enroll in a clinical study, you should talk with both your urologist and oncologist about the specifics of the potential study as well as have a full understanding of the potential risks and benefits to you. Compare these potential

Randomized

the process of assigning patients to different forms of treatment in a research study in a random manner.

Food and Drug Administration

the agency responsible for the approval of prescription medications in the United States.

Metastatic Disease

risks and benefits carefully to the standard, proven therapy being offered by your doctors (see the appendix for Internet addresses of sites that list clinical trials and provide more information for those patients interested in pursuing clinical trials).

PART EIGHT

End-of-Life Care

I have never thought of dying before, but now that I have been diagnosed with bladder cancer, I find myself wondering, are there things that I should do to prepare for death?

If aggressive treatment is too much to bear or seems futile, is it okay to stop treating my cancer?

More . . .

98. I have never thought of dying before, but now that I have been diagnosed with bladder cancer, I find myself wondering, are there things that I should do to prepare for death?

None of us likes to think about the end of life, particularly while we still feel young and healthy. Many of us are poorly prepared to think about dying. As a result, many people have not made appropriate preparations with their families, physicians, lawyers, and so forth. End-of-life decisions, such as **living wills**, healthcare proxies, and **advanced directives** should be addressed directly long before you become ill and potentially unable to communicate your wishes.

If you have never had a serious discussion with your family about your views on the end of life, now is the time. For many American families, this can be a difficult discussion, but it is important to persist. By the end of the discussion, your family should be able to verbalize your feelings on several issues. First, if you were to stop breathing on your own, would you want to be placed on a ventilator if there were a good chance that you could eventually come off the ventilator and breathe on your own? What if there was not a good chance of coming off the ventilator? Second, if your heart were to stop beating, would you want to have CPR and/or defibrillation (shocking with "the paddles")? Third, if you were unable to eat on your own, would you want to be fed through a tube in your stomach? Fourth, if you are unable to communicate with your doctors, who should be your voice to make decisions about your health care? You should choose a single family member or close friend if no family member

Living will

a document in which you can state specific instructions regarding your health care, including measures that would prolong your life; it may outline which medical interventions you want to have performed and which you want to have withheld for a variety of circumstances.

Advanced directives

legal documents in which you indicate who you want to make medical decisions for you and/or what type of medical care you want to receive if you become unable to make decisions or speak for yourself.

is able or willing to act on your behalf. It is important that everyone in your family be aware of your choice and is accepting of it. Legally, your spouse is first in line to make decisions followed by adult children, although most states will allow you to choose if you fill out and sign the appropriate forms.

Once your family understands your feelings and directives about end-of-life care, you should think about how those who depend on you would get along if you were not there. If you are in charge of the finances, you need to show someone where all your records are kept and counsel that person as to how to manage the finances in your absence. Similarly, any other chore or duty that is exclusively yours needs to be addressed.

For most of us, it can be helpful to consult an estate-planning attorney to guide us through the legal process associated with these decisions. The American Cancer Society has a brochure that discusses the common issues that should be addressed, including questions regarding business, taxes, and loans. You will want to make sure that the following are in order: life insurance, retirement plans, titles to assets, property, bank accounts, safe deposit boxes, stocks, bonds, car deeds, and your will. It is important that beneficiaries are clearly designated and that account numbers, addresses, telephone numbers, and contact information are recorded. All of this information needs to be kept somewhere that is easily accessible to your family, and your family should know that you have taken care of these things for them.

99. If aggressive treatment is too much to bear or seems futile, is it okay to stop treating my cancer?

The most basic credo of modern medicine is "first, do no harm." Many of the treatments that we now have available, although often lifesaving, can be painful or difficult for patients and their families. We offer these treatments and encourage patients to persist because we truly believe that after all is said and done, the patient will be better off for it. Unfortunately, we are still not able to cure everyone, and some patients eventually may be faced with little or no chance of real benefit from ongoing treatments. To continue with aggressive treatment can be physically and emotionally painful at a time when the patient would be better served by improving his or her life rather than extending it. Although these situations are difficult for doctors, patients, and their families, it is important that everyone be honest and open. Ultimately, it should always be the patient's decision whether to continue treatment or to move to what is called **palliative** therapy.

Palliative

treatment designed to relieve a particular problem without necessarily solving it; for example, palliative therapy is given to relieve symptoms and improve quality of life, but it does not cure the patient.

Palliative therapy is designed to provide a patient with the best quality of life possible without regard to long-term cure of a terminal disease. Choosing palliative care does not mean that you have chosen *no* care. Although the specific treatments that you choose to accept will be specific your situation, most patients will still receive blood transfusions when needed, radiation treatments aimed at reducing bone pain, medications, and even surgery if it would improve bothersome symptoms. Choosing palliative care means an acceptance that your cancer is incurable, but it allows you to continue receiving certain treatments.

Palliative therapy is somewhat different than care termed "comfort measures only." Patients who have chosen to limit their treatments to comfort measures only usually have very little time to live and will essentially receive only pain medications to keep them comfortable. They would usually not receive blood transfusions or dialysis, undergo surgery, and the like.

Dealing with my mother's death was difficult. She had always been very clear that she did not want to be on a ventilator or feeding tubes, that she wanted to maintain her dignity if the outcome was clear. When she was doing well, it seemed like it would be easy to follow her wishes. But they never come to you and say clearly that "this is the moment" to let her go. There's always another treatment, another doctor, another something. It was easy to make the decision to provide palliative care only because mom could still speak for herself. The "comfort measures only" decision placed much more responsibility on the family. After long discussions with her doctors, we finally agreed that keeping her comfortable and allowing her to rest peacefully would be the best way to honor her life and her wishes. It helped that we had all been able to talk openly with my mother about the end while she was well, and I know it was what she would have wanted, but it was still the hardest decision I've ever had to make. (M. D., 59 years old)

100. What is hospice care?

Hospice care is designed to provide care to patients at the end of life. The term originates from the same root as "hospitality," the idea of providing shelter to a sick or weary traveler. According to the American Cancer

Hospice

a program that provides care to patients at the end of their life; can be provided at home or at an inpatient facility.

Society, "Hospice provides humane and compassionate care for people in the last phases of incurable disease so that they may live as fully and comfortably as possible. . . . It seeks to enable patients to continue an alert, pain-free life and to manage other symptoms so that their last days may be spent with dignity and quality, surrounded by their loved ones." To qualify for hospice care, a physician must deem the patient "terminal." This designation is legally defined as "a six-month life expectancy assuming the disease runs its normal course." Hospice care is usually provided in a patient's home, although it may also be provided in a nursing home, hospital, or private hospice facility. If your condition improves or you would prefer to again receive more aggressive treatments, you can be discharged from hospice care at any time with the option of returning in the future. For more details about the types of hospice care available, call the American Cancer Society or see their web site at *www.cancer.org*.

Appendix

Organizations

American Cancer Society
1599 Clifton Road
Atlanta, GA 30329
www.cancer.org
1-800-ACS-2345

American Foundation for Urologic Disease
300 West Pratt Street
Suite 401
Baltimore, MD 21201-2463
www.afud.org
1-800-242-2383

American Society of Clinical Oncology
1900 Duke Street
Suite 200
Alexandria, VA 22314
www.asco.org
703-299-0150

National Cancer Institute
National Cancer Institute Public Information Office
Building 31, Room 10A31
31 Center Drive, MSC 2580
Bethesda, MD 20892-2580
www.nci.nih.gov
301-435-3848

Web Sites with General Cancer Information

411Cancer.com
About.com (search on "cancer")
CancerLinks.org
CancerSource.com
CancerWiseTM/MD/Anderson Cancer Center, *www.cancer-wise.org*
National Cancer Institute's CancerNet Service, *cancernet.nci.nih.gov/index.html*
Medicalconsumerguide.com
Acor.org

Web Pages on Specific Topics

Chemotherapy
www.yana.org offers online and in-person support groups for those going through high-dose chemotherapy.
Drug information for chemotherapy, including information on financial assistance *www.cancersupportivecare.com/pharmacy.html*

Clinical Trials

The National Cancer Institute's Cancer Trials site lists current clinical trials that have been reviewed by the National Cancer Institute.

Coping

The National Coalition for Cancer Survivorship (*www.cancersearch.org*, phone: 877-NCCS-YES) offers a free audio program, "Cancer Survivor Toolbox," including ways to cope with the illness (the web site also has a newsletter, requiring a yearly membership fee).

R.A. Bloch Cancer Foundation (*www.blochcancer.org*) offers an inspirational online book about cancer, relaxation techniques, and positive outlooks on fighting cancer, as well as trained one-on-one support from fellow cancer patients.

Diet and Nutrition (Cancer Prevention)/USDA Dietary guidelines are listed at *www.usda.gov/cnpp*.

American Institute for Cancer Research provides tips on how to reduce cancer risk (*www.aicr.org*).

Cancer Research Foundation of America's healthy eating suggestions (*www.preventcancer.org/whdiet.cfm*).

Family Resources

This web site (*www.kidscope.org*) is designed to help children understand and deal with the effects of cancer on a parent.

Legal Protections, Financial Resources, and Insurance Coverage

The American Cancer Society offers a number of relevant documents to help you understand your coverage, legal protections, and how to find financial assistance. Search *http://www.cancer.org* using the keyword "insurance."

Medicaid information can be found at *http://www.hcfa.gov/medical/medicaid.htm*.

"Every question you need to ask before selling your life insurance policy" is by the National Viator Representatives, Inc. Call 1-800-932-0050 for a free copy or go to *www.nvrnvr.com*.

Family and Medical Leave Act can be seen at *www.dol.gov/dol/esa/public/regs/statutes/whd/fmla.htm*.

This web site, *www.needymeds.com*, offers information about programs sponsored by pharmaceutical manufacturers to help people who cannot afford to purchase necessary drugs.

This web site, *www.cancercare.org/hhrd/hhrd_financial.htm*, offers listings of where to look for financial assistance.

The National Financial Resource Book For Patients: a state-by-state directory is found at *data.patientadvocate.org/*.

Glossary

Abdomen: The part of the body that is below the ribs and above the pelvic bone; it contains organs such as the intestines, the liver, the kidneys, the bladder, and the prostate.

Abscess: A localized collection of pus in part of the body.

Adenocarcinoma: A form of cancer that develops from a malignant abnormality in the cells lining a glandular organ; a less common form of cancer of the bladder.

Advanced directives: Legal documents in which you indicate who you want to make medical decisions for you and/or what type of medical care you want to receive if you become unable to make decisions or speak for yourself.

Anesthesia: The loss of feeling or sensation; with respect to surgery, the loss of sensation of pain, as it is induced to allow surgery or other painful procedures to be performed. General anesthesia is a state of unconsciousness, produced by anes-

thetic agents, with absence of pain sensation over the entire body and a greater or lesser degree of muscle relaxation. Local anesthesia is confined to one part of the body. Spinal anesthesia is produced by injection of a local anesthetic into the subarachnoid space around the spinal cord.

Aniline dyes: A class of synthetic, organic dyes obtained from aniline (coal tars). These dyes have been used to impart color to paper, cloth, and leather, and have been used in woodworking.

Attenuated: To reduce in force, value, amount, or degree; to weaken. With respect to a bacteria/virus, to reduce the infectivity of a pathogenic microorganism.

BCG: As it pertains to bladder cancer, live attenuated tuberculosis bacteria that are placed into the bladder (intravesical therapy) to decrease the recurrence of bladder cancer.

Benign: A noncancerous tumor that can expand and press on surrounding structures but does not invade them and does not spread to a distant site.

Biopsy: The removal of small sample(s) of tissue for examination under the microscope.

Bladder: The hollow organ that stores and discharges urine from the body.

BTA: A protein found in bladder cancer cells but not in normal cells. A urine test is available to check for BTA.

Cancer: Abnormal and uncontrolled growth of cells in the body that may spread, injure areas of the body, and lead to death.

Carcinoma: A form of cancer that originates in tissues that line or cover a particular organ.

Carcinoma in situ: Pertaining to bladder cancer, a superficial-appearing bladder cancer associated with a high risk of subsequent invasive disease.

Cardiovascular disease: Disease of the heart or blood vessels.

Catheter: A hollow tube that allows for fluid drainage from or injection into an area.

Cautery: The application of a caustic substance—a hot instrument, an electric current, or other agent—to destroy tissue or control bleeding.

Cell: The smallest unit of the body. Tissues in the body are made of cells.

Cellulitis: An inflammation/infection of the skin and underlying tissue presenting with a warm, red swollen area.

Cervix: The lower, narrow end of the uterus that connects to the vagina.

Chemotherapy: A treatment for cancer that uses powerful medications to weaken and destroy the cancer cells.

Chronic obstructive pulmonary disease: A progressive disease that most commonly results from smoking, characterized by difficulty breathing, wheezing, and a chronic cough.

Clinical trials: A carefully planned experiment to evaluate a treatment or medication (often a new drug) for an unproven use.

Collecting system: As it pertains to the kidney, the renal pelvis and calyces.

Colostomy: The surgical construction of an "atypical anus" between the colon and the surface of the abdomen.

Complication: An undesirable result of a treatment, surgery, or medication.

Conduit: A method of diverting the urine flow by sewing the ureters—the tubes that drain the kidneys—to a segment of intestine that is closed at one end. The open end is sewn to the abdominal wall to allow for urine to drain into a collecting bag.

Continence: With respect to urine, the ability to retain urine until the proper time to release it.

Continent urinary diversion: A form of urinary diversion enabling one to store urine. The urine is emptied several times a day by placing a catheter into a small channel that connects the conduit to the abdominal wall and allows the urine to drain through the catheter.

CT scan (computerized tomography/computerized axial tomography): A specialized X-ray study that allows one to visualize internal structures in cross-section to look for abnormalities.

Cystectomy: Removal of the bladder. Partial cystectomy is removal of a portion of the bladder. Radical cystectomy involves removal of the bladder—in males, the prostate and seminal vesicles and in females, the uterus and cervix.

Cystitis: Inflammation of the bladder; may be related to a bacterial infection, viral infection, radiation, or other bladder irritants.

Cystoscope: A telescope-like instrument that allows examination of the urethra and the inside of the bladder.

Cystoscopy: The procedure of using a cystoscope to look into the urethra and bladder.

Cytology: The study of cells under a microscope.

Day surgery: Refers to a surgical procedure that is performed on the day of surgery the patient goes home that same day. It does not require an overnight hospitalization. It is also called outpatient surgery.

Deep venous thrombosis: Blood clotting in the veins of the inner thigh or leg.

Diagnosis: The identification of the cause or presence of a medical problem or disease.

Disease: Any change from or interruption of the normal structure or function of any part or organ system of the body, presenting characteristic symptoms and signs whose cause and prognosis may be known or unknown.

Diverticulum: In the bladder, a small sac-like structure that lacks a muscular coat and thus does not contract like other areas of the bladder.

DNA: The basic building block of cells. It carries the cell's genetic information and hereditary characteristics.

Dyspareunia: Difficult or painful coitus (sex).

Dysplasia: An alteration in the size, shape, and organization of adult cells.

Dysuria: Pain or discomfort with urination.

Efficacy: The power or ability to produce an effect.

Epidermal growth factor: A chemical that stimulates growth of cells.

Epididymis: A structure attached to the testes that stores sperm as they mature. Epididymis connects to the vas deferens.

Epithelial cells: Cells that cover the surface of the body and line its cavities.

Erectile dysfunction: The inability to achieve and/or maintain an erection satisfactory for the completion of sexual performance.

Experimental: An untested or unproven treatment or approach to treatment.

Fallopian tubes: Two long muscular tubes that transport ova (eggs) from the ovaries to the uterus.

Fascia: A fibrous membrane covering, supporting, and separating muscles.

FISH—fluorescent in situ hybridization: A test that looks directly at the DNA of a cell to identify malignant cells.

Fistulae: Abnormal passages or communication between two internal organs or leading from an internal organ to the surface of the body.

Foley catheter: A catheter that is placed into the bladder via the urethra to drain urine.

Food and Drug Administration (FDA): The agency responsible for the approval of prescription medications in the United States.

Frequency: The need to urinate often. In adults, it is often used to describe the need to urinate eight or more times per day.

Gallbladder: A digestive tract organ that stores bile, a chemical produced in the liver.

Genes: Located in the nucleus of the cell, genes contain hereditary information that is transferred from cell to cell.

Genetics: A field of medicine that studies heredity.

Grade: With respect to tumors, an assessment of the aggressiveness of the tumor by how the cells look under the microscope.

Hematuria: The presence of blood in the urine. It may be gross (visible) or microscopic (only detected under the microscope).

Hernia: A weakening in the muscle that leads to a bulge.

High grade: Very advanced cancer cells.

High risk: More likely to have a complication or side effect.

History: An oral or written interview that consists of questions about your medical, social, and family background.

Hospice: A program that provides care to patients at the end of their life, provided at home or at an inpatient facility.

Hydronephrosis: Dilation of the renal pelvis and calyces of one or both kidneys because of accumulation of urine resulting from obstruction of the outflow of urine.

Hysterectomy: Removal of the uterus.

Ileal conduit: A form of urinary diversion that uses a piece of small intestine as the conduit.

Ileum: A part of the small intestine.

Immune response: The body's response to things it identifies as foreign or not normal.

Immune system: The body system, made up of many organs and cells, that defends the body against infection, disease, and foreign substances. The immune system is often stimulated in specific ways to fight cancer cells.

Immunocompromised: A condition in which the immune system is not functioning properly.

ImmunoCyt: A urine test for bladder cancer. It checks for three different proteins at the same time.

Immunotherapy: Therapy designed to activate the body's own immune system to fight disease.

Incarcerated: With respect to bowel, bowel that is trapped, and may lead to swelling and decreased blood flow to the bowel segment.

Incidence: The rate at which a certain event occurs, for example, the number of new cases of a specific disease occurring during a certain period.

Incision: Cutting of the skin at the beginning of surgery.

Incontinence: The involuntary loss of urine.

Indication: The reason for undertaking a specific treatment.

Inflammation: Swelling, redness, pain, and irritation as the result of injury, infection, or surgery.

In situ: In the natural or normal place.

Interferon: A substance produced by cells that suppresses the growth of cells and regulates the immune response.

Interventional radiologist: A radiologist who specializes in minimally invasive, targeted treatments performed using imaging for guidance.

Intravenous: Into the veins.

Intravenous pyelogram: A radiologic study in which a dye is injected into the veins and is picked up by the kidneys and passed out into the urine. It allows one to visualize the urinary tract.

Intravesical therapy: Medical therapy that is placed into the bladder to kill cancer cells. The therapy is placed into the bladder through a urethral catheter.

Invasive: In cancer, the spread of the cancer beyond the site where it initially developed into surrounding tissues.

Irritative voiding symptoms: The symptoms of urinary frequency and urgency.

Laparoscope: A specialized telescope-like device that allows one to see into the abdominal cavity and pelvis through a very small incision.

Laparoscopy: An operation that uses a laparoscope and other modified equipment that may be passed through very small incisions in the abdominal wall.

Libido: Sexual desire, interest in sex.

Lifestyle: The way a person chooses to live.

Living will: A document in which you can state specific instructions regarding your health care, including measures that would prolong your life; may outline which medical interventions you want to have performed and which you want to have withheld for a variety of circumstances.

Locally advanced: Describes when a cancerous tumor has spread to surrounding structures.

Low grade: Cancer that does not appear aggressive, advanced.

Lymph node: A small bean-shaped organ that is part of the immune system; nodes filter out bacteria or cancer cells that may travel though the lymphatic system.

Lymphocele: A collection of lymph fluid in an area of the body.

Lymphatic system: The tissues and organs (the bone marrow, spleen, thymus, and lymph nodes) that produce and store cells that fight infection and the network of vessels that carry lymph.

Magnetic resonance imaging: A study similar to a CT scan in that it allows someone to see internal structures in detail, but it does not involve radiation.

Malignant: A cancerous tumor; can invade surrounding structures and spread to a distant site.

Metastasis: The transfer of disease (cancer cells) from one organ or part to another not directly connected with it.

Metastasize: Describes when a cancerous tumor has spread to a distant site, for example, the bones, the liver, or the brain.

Microscopic: Small enough that a microscope is needed to see it.

Mitomycin C: A chemical that prevents the production of DNA and that prevents cell growth.

Morbidity: Unhealthy results and complications resulting from treatment.

Nasogastric tube: A tube placed through the nose down the esophagus into the stomach to drain fluid accumulating in the stomach.

Negative: A test result that does not show what one is looking for.

Neobladder: An artificial/new bladder, created by using a portion of the intestines, that stores urine like a real bladder and allows one to urinate per urethra.

Nephrostomy tube: A tube placed through the back into the kidney that allows for drainage of urine from that kidney.

Nerve: A cord-like structure composed of a collection of nerve fibers that conveys impulses between a part of the central nervous system and some other region of the body.

Nerve-sparing surgery: A surgical procedure for men with prostate or bladder cancer in which the prostate or bladder is removed and the nerves are left undisturbed with the goal of preserving erectile function.

NMP 22: A protein that undergoes changes when a bladder cell becomes cancerous. A urine test has been developed that tests for these changes in NMP 22.

Noninvasive: Not requiring any incision or the insertion of an instrument or substance into the body.

Obstruction: The state or condition of being blocked/clogged.

Obturator nerve: A nerve located on the pelvis that produces motor innervation to muscles in the thigh and skin sensation to the inner thigh.

Oncogenes: Genes that can potentially induce neoplastic transformation (development of cancer).

Oncologist: A physician who specializes in treating cancer. Urologic oncologists specialize in surgical therapy for cancers of the genitourinary tract. Medical oncologists specialize in treatment with chemotherapy, hormonal therapy, and biologic therapy; and radiation oncologists specialize in treating with radiation.

Oral: Taken by mouth.

Organ: Tissues in the body (i.e., heart, bladder) that work together to perform a specific function.

Orthotopic: In the normal or usual position.

Ostomy bag: A specialized bag that is applied over an ostomy to collect urine and stool.

Overactive bladder: A syndrome with symptoms of urgency, frequency, nocturia, and sometimes urge incontinence. It is thought to be related to overactivity of the bladder muscle.

p21 ras oncogene: A specialized oncogene that has been associated with cancers in humans.

Palliative: Treatment designed to relieve a particular problem without necessarily solving it; for example, palliative therapy is given to relieve symptoms and improve quality of life, but it does not cure the patient.

Papillary: Related to bladder cancer, a bladder cancer that has a stalk with nipple-like projections.

Parasite: An organism that obtains food and shelter from another organism.

Pathologist: A doctor trained in the evaluation of tissues under the microscope to determine the presence or absence of disease.

Pathology: The branch of medicine concerned with disease, especially its structure and functional effects on the body.

Pelvic lymph node dissection: In the case of bladder cancer, pelvic lymph node dissection, which is the surgical removal of the lymph nodes in the pelvis to determine whether the bladder cancer has spread to these nodes.

Pelvis: The part of the body that is framed by the hip bones.

Perioperative chemotherapy: Chemotherapy administered shortly before planned surgery in hopes of improving local control and survival.

Photodynamic therapy: Cancer treatment that uses the interaction between laser light and a substance that makes cells more sensitive to light. When light is applied to cells that have been treated with this substance, a chemical reaction occurs and destroys cancer cells.

Photosensitizer: An agent that makes the tissue photosensitive when applied or absorbed.

Postvoid residual: The volume of urine left in the bladder at the end of micturition.

Premalignant (precancerous): In a very early stage of cancer development; abnormal changes occur in tissue as a predeterminant for possible future malignancy.

Prognosis: The long-term outlook or prospect for survival and recovery from a disease.

Progression: The continued growth of cancer or disease.

Prophylactic: Preventive measure or medication.

Prostate: A gland within the male reproductive system that is located just below the bladder surrounding part of the urethra, the canal that empties the bladder; produces a fluid that forms part of semen.

Prostatitis: Inflammation of the prostate; may be infectious or inflammatory.

Prosthetics: The art and science of making and adjusting artificial parts of the human body.

Proteins: Any group of complex organic macromolecules that contain carbon, hydrogen, oxygen, nitrogen, and usually sulfur and are composed of alpha-amino acids. Proteins are fundamental components of all living cells and include many substances such as enzymes, hormones, and antibodies that are necessary to the functioning of an organism.

Protocol: Research study used to evaluate a specific medication or treatment.

Pulmonary embolism: The obstruction of pulmonary arteries (arteries in the lungs), usually by detached fragments of a clot from a leg or pelvic vein.

Pyelonephritis: Infection of the kidney, most commonly bacterial in origin.

Pyridium: A medication that acts as a urinary tract anesthetic. It turns the urine an orange color.

Quality of life: An evaluation of healthy status relative to the patient's age, expectations, and physical and mental capabilities.

Radiation: The application of energy in the form of rays or waves to treat various medical conditions.

Radiation oncologist: A physician who treats cancer through the use of radiation therapy.

Radiation therapy: The use of high-energy radiation to destroy cancer cells; also called radiotherapy or irradiation.

Randomized: The process of assigning patients to different forms of treatment in a research study in a random manner.

Rectum: The last portion of the large intestine that communicates with the sigmoid colon above and the anus below.

Recurrence: The reappearance of disease.

Renal pelvis: The area at the center of the kidney. Urine collects in the renal pelvis and is funneled into the ureter.

Resected: Removed surgically.

Resectoscope: A specialized cystoscope-like device that is passed through the urethra through which one may remove bladder tumors by using a loop device connected to an electrical current.

Retrograde pyelogram: A specialized study to look at the ureter and collecting system of the kidney; involves placement of a tube into the ureteral orifice and injecting contrast/dye.

Rhabdomyosarcoma: A malignant tumor derived from striated skeletal muscle.

Risk: The chance or probability that a particular event will or will not happen.

Salpingo-oophorectomy: Removal of the fallopian tube and ovary; may be unilateral or bilateral.

Salvage: A procedure intended to "rescue" a patient after a failed prior therapy.

Schistosomiasis: A parasite that is a "fluke" or "worm." The parasite first infects fresh water snails, and then the larvae are released into the water and can penetrate unbroken skin of humans. The parasite can then infect the liver, intestine, bladder, kidneys, or lung. Infection of the bladder can lead to bladder cancer. Schistosomiasis is found in sub-Saharan Africa, Southern China, the Philippines, Brazil, and Egypt.

Seminal vesicles: Paired glandular structures that are located above and behind the prostate gland. They produce fluid that is part of the ejaculate. They are removed during a radical cystectomy.

Sensitivity: The probability that a diagnostic test can correctly identify the presence of a particular disease.

Serosa: One of the delicate membranes of connective tissue that line the internal cavities of the body.

Sessile: Pertaining to bladder cancer, a cancer that is broad-based and stalkless.

Side effect: A reaction to a medication or treatment.

Sign: Objective evidence of a disease or condition; that is, something the doctor identifies.

Slow acetylator: Someone who metabolizes certain chemicals slower than others do.

Squamous cell carcinoma: Of the bladder, a type of cancer that typically occurs in chronically inflamed bladders, such as in individuals with chronic indwelling catheters.

Stage: A measure of how extensive the cancer is and how much it has spread.

Staging: The process of determining the extent of disease. It is helpful in determining the most appropriate treatment. It often involves physical examination, blood testing, and X-ray studies.

Stoma: A surgically created opening in the skin for elimination of body waste, such as urine or stool.

Stomal stenoses: Narrowing of the stoma.

Straining to void: The muscular effort used to either initiate, maintain, or improve the flow of urine.

Stricture: Scarring as a result of a procedure or an injury that causes narrowing.

Superficial: Near the surface.

Symptom: Subjective evidence of a disease, that is, something that the patient describes, such as pain in the abdomen.

Testicle: The male reproductive organ that produces testosterone and sperm. Normally, there are 2 located in the scrotum.

Thiotepa: A form of chemotherapy used intravesically for bladder cancer.

Tissue: Specific type of material in the body, for example muscle, hair.

TNM: A specialized cancer-staging system that assesses the extent of cancer in the organ in which the cancer developed, the lymph nodes, and surrounding/distant tissues/organs.

Total parenteral nutrition: An intravenous form of nutrition that provides all essential nutrients.

Transurethral resection of bladder tumor (TURBT): Removal of a bladder tumor(s) though a specialized instrument, a resectoscope, that is passed through the penis into the bladder.

Tumor: An abnormal swelling or mass.

Tumor suppressor genes: A group of genes that act to slow down the growth/development of a cancer/tumor.

Ultrasound: A technique used to look at internal organs by measuring reflected sound waves.

Upper tract study: A radiologic study used to evaluate the kidneys and ureters.

Urachal carcinoma: Cancer that develops in the urachus. Although classified as a bladder cancer, this cancer develops outside of the bladder and grows into the bladder.

Urachal ligament: The remnant of the urachus.

Urachus: The urinary canal of the fetus. In the fetus, it communicates with the bladder and the umbilicus. After birth, it is usually a fibrous cord.

Ureteral orifice: The terminal opening of the ureter, normally located in the bladder.

Ureteral stent: A plastic tube used to keep the ureter open and allow for the drainage of urine.

Ureteroscope: A long, slender cystoscope-like device that allows one to visualize the ureter, renal pelvis, and calyces.

Ureterosigmoidostomy: A specialized procedure whereby the ureters are connected to the sigmoid colon. Urine is thus evacuated with stools.

Ureterostomy: Surgical formation of an opening in the ureter for external drainage of the urine; in a cutaneous ureterostomy, ureteral orifice is brought through the abdominal wall on the skin.

Ureters: Muscular tubes that connect the kidneys to the bladder, through which urine passes into the bladder.

Urethra: The tube through which one urinates.

Urgency: The complaint of a sudden compelling desire to void that is difficult to defer.

Urinary diversion: A surgical procedure that diverts the flow of urine away from the bladder, typically to the abdominal wall, either directly by sewing the ureters to the skin or more commonly by sewing the ureters to a conduit; see **conduit**.

Urinary retention: The inability to urinate, leading to a filled bladder.

Urinary tract infection: Infection of the urinary tract with microorganisms. It may involve the bladder (cystitis) and/or the kidney (pyelon-ephritis).

Urine cytology: A test that is performed by a specialized pathologist (cytopathologist) whereby the urine is examined for the presence of abnormal cells suggestive or characteristic of cancer cells.

Urologist: A doctor who specializes in the evaluation and treatment of diseases of the genitourinary tract in males and females.

Urostomy: A conduit for the drainage of urine from the kidneys to the anterior abdominal wall. May be made from small or large intestine.

Urostomy bag: A specialized collecting device applied to the urostomy stoma that collects urine.

Urothelium: The cells lining the wall of the bladder, ureter, and the collecting system of the kidney.

Uterus: The muscular pelvic organ of the female reproductive system in which the fetus develops.

Valsalva voiding: Use of abdominal muscles to increase bladder pressure to empty the bladder during voiding.

Vas deferens: A tubular structure that connects the epididymus to the urethea, through which sperm and seminal fluid passes.

Index

Index